Foods That Cause You To Lose Weight

The Negative Calorie Effect

by Neal Barnard, M.D.

Recipes adapted from *Judy Brown's Guide to Natural Foods
Cooking*, by Judy Brown and Dorothy R. Bates

Interior design by Barbara McNew
Printed in U.S.A.

0 9 8 7 6 5 4 3 2
ISBN 1-882330-00-5

Table of Contents

Introduction

This book offers a new approach to weight control. If your goal is a slimmer body and more energy than you have had in years, this program is more powerful than any diet you have ever tried. It is not a diet. It is a comprehensive program that brings about better weight control than old-fashioned diets ever could.

In this program, we will not compromise. We will use all the factors that are known to promote permanent healthful weight control. You will boost your metabolic rate through food selection, shift your menu from calorie-dense fatty foods to foods with a much better nutrient make-up, and bring in other ways to burn calories more effectively.

This book was written because most diets have not been very successful. Many are simply too weak to get results. Others use an artificial "formula approach" that no one could live with permanently. They may cause a phenomenal weight loss for a few weeks, followed by a huge weight gain back to and beyond the starting point. These frustrating results are caused by the poor design of the diets.

There is a much better way. For years, researchers have used many different kinds of diets to improve health: diets to help people lose weight, lower their cholesterol levels, or deal with various health problems. From these studies, it is clear that there are certain factors which are critical to success in long-term weight control.

For example:

✦ Certain foods add easily to fat stores while others do not.
✦ Certain foods will alter your metabolism so that calories are burned more effectively.
✦ Weight loss should be gradual, not sudden.
✦ And, most importantly, a menu that is very low in fat, high in fiber and carbohydrate, and modest in protein, is extraordinarily powerful for weight control.

We will examine these and many other factors in detail.

Old diets focused mainly on quantity. In the new approach used in this program, the type of food that makes up the menu is considerably more important than the quantity of food. In other words, *you can eat until you are full and still lose weight*. No more skimpy portions. If you find that difficult to believe, consider the research. Many clinical studies have examined diets that are based on very small portions and other diets that change the type of food but not the quantity. It turns out that *the type of food you eat is much more important for permanent weight control than the portion size*. In fact, skimpy portion diets can actually impair your ability to burn off calories. Research also shows that thin people actually eat more food, not less, compared to most overweight people. In this program, we will shift the diet toward foods that boost the metabolism and which do not easily add to body fat.

There are also specific factors that make the process of change easier. A diet that brings about long-term success is much more rewarding than one that yields only modest or short-term results. So this program is designed to be as effective as possible.

We will also have opportunities to try new kinds of foods. This is not only fun; it is the critical step in building a new body. Tasting food is when theories about weight control turn into practice. You will learn about specific new foods to try, including menus, recipes, and shopping lists. In addition, we will look at ways to bring in family and friends. They are our allies in life's changes. We will see how to help them help us.

When you put this program to work for you, you can have the slimmest body nature ever intended for you.

How to Use This Program

This program is divided into four parts:

Basic Concepts	First, find a comfortable chair and read Part One. In this concise section, you will learn the basic concepts that are essential to a permanent slimming-down program.
Step-by-Step Program	Part Two gets you started with a step-by-step program, including new foods to try, and recipes, and a simple program for physical activity. You can easily chart your progress.
Keeping It Off	Part Three moves the program into high gear, with more advanced information to solidify your gains.
Menus & Recipes	Part Four gives you many more healthful recipes to make eating a joy.

Get all you can out of this program. No corners were cut in bringing this information to you; do not cut any corners in putting it into action.

You can succeed. So be patient, and don't rush. It took time for you to gain weight, and it will take time for it to come off again. Overly rapid weight loss can lead to a rebound of weight gain, so let the pounds come off gradually. I think you will be happy with the new you.

Notice

This book is not intended to take the place of medical advice.

✦ If you have any medical condition or are on medication, you should consult your doctor before making any substantial change in your diet. Dietary changes can sometimes change your need for medication or have other important effects.

✦ You should also see your doctor before any substantial increase in your physical activity if you are over forty or have any medical condition.

✦ If you are pregnant or nursing, or if you follow this program strictly for more than three years, then take 3 micrograms supplemental vitamin B_{12} each day.

Part I

Basic Concepts

Basic Concepts

We need to think differently about the approach to losing weight. Forget old-fashioned diets. There are very good reasons why they do not work well. Your body was not designed recently. The human body took shape millions of years ago, long before diets were invented. At that time, the lack of food meant only one thing, starvation; and if the body could not cope with the lack of food, the result was life-threatening. So we have built-in mechanisms to preserve ourselves in the face of low food intake. These defenses are automatically put to work. When you go on a low-calorie diet, you know that you are doing so to lose weight. But your body does not know that. As far as your body is concerned you are starving, and it will trigger a number of biological mechanisms to try and stop you.

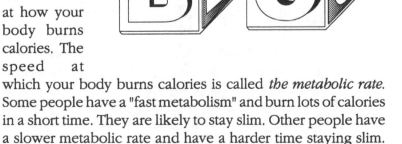

To see how to avoid this problem, let's first look at how your body burns calories. The speed at which your body burns calories is called *the metabolic rate*. Some people have a "fast metabolism" and burn lots of calories in a short time. They are likely to stay slim. Other people have a slower metabolic rate and have a harder time staying slim.

Your metabolism is like the rate at which an automobile uses up gas. An idling car uses up some fuel. When the car is moving it uses more, and when it accelerates up a hill it will use a lot more gas.

Our bodies work the same way. We burn some calories even when we are relaxing or asleep because it takes energy to maintain our normal body temperature and to keep our lungs, heart, brain and other organs working. When we engage in activities, the more strenuous they are, the more calories we burn.

Dieting Slows Your Metabolism

The point to remember is that your metabolic rate can be changed. In a period of starvation or dieting, the body slows down the metabolism. The body does not understand the concept of dieting. Remember, as far as your body is concerned, a diet is starvation, and it does not know how long the starvation period will last. So it clings to its fat like a motorist who is running out of gas preserves fuel. Remember the last time you were driving along the highway and suddenly noticed that the gas gauge was below empty? You tried to remember how far below "E" your gauge will go. You went easy on the accelerator, driving very smoothly, and turned off the engine at stop lights to conserve gas until you got to a station.

Your body does the same sort of thing when food is in short supply. It turns down the metabolic flame to save as much of the fat on your body as possible until the starvation period is over, because fat is the body's fuel reserve. This is very frustrating to dieters. They often find that, even though they are eating very little, their bodies do not easily shed the pounds. Even worse, the slowed metabolism can continue beyond the dieting period, sometimes for weeks, according to studies at the University of Pennsylvania and elsewhere.[1] For that reason, fat is easily and rapidly accumulated again after the dieting period. This causes the familiar yo-yo phenomenon, in which dieters lose some weight, then rebound to a higher weight than they started with.

Here is the first step to keeping your metabolic rate up: Make sure that your diet contains at least 10 calories per pound of your ideal body weight. This means that if you are aiming for a weight of 150 pounds, your daily menu should contain at least 1500 calories. Weight loss will be gradual, but you will not slow your metabolism and, so, you will be able to retain your progress.

Minimum Calories per day

Ideal Weight x 10 calories = Calories

120 x 10 calories = 1200 Calories
150 x 10 calories = 1500 Calories
180 x 10 calories = 1800 Calories

Avoiding Binges

There is another problem with skimpy eating. Not only does the body lower its metabolic flame to conserve energy; it also gets ready to take maximal advantage of any food source it finds. When food becomes available, there is a tremendous tendency to binge, in what is known as the "*restrained-eater*" phenomenon. You know the pattern. You have been dieting for several days, and suddenly someone brings home a carton of ice cream. A little bit won't hurt, you decide, and before you know it you are scraping the bottom of the carton and digging around the cracks for every last bit. You then scold yourself for your "lack of

The point to remember is binges come from diets.

will power." The truth is that the problem was not will power at all, but, rather, the innate biological programming of the human body. The diet turned on the "anti-starvation" plan that is built into every human being. Your body assumed that any food in front of you might be the only calorie source you might have for a while, so it demanded a binge.

It is not a question of weak will or gluttony. The human body has a built-in tendency to binge after periods of starvation.

For a similar reason, it is best not to skip meals. Skipping breakfast and lunch leads to overeating later in the day. So, eat regular meals and avoid very-low-calorie diets.

Bulimia—binge-eating often followed by purging—almost always begins with a diet. And as the binging begins, shame and secrecy often follow. If this has happened to you, remember that binging is not a moral failing. It is a natural biological consequence of dieting.

Dieting is now a nearly universal pastime in America, and bulimia is an ever-growing epidemic. Unfortunately, children are raised on a menu that is almost certain to make many of them gain weight. The cultural trend in Western countries in the past several decades has emphasized meat, dairy products, fried; chicken, french fries and other high-fat foods. Combined with an increasingly sedentary lifestyle, the predictable result is that many people will become overweight. They mistakenly believe that the problem is the *quantity* of food they are eating, rather than the *type* of food. Rather than abandon the offending foods, they simply eat less. A restrictive diet begins. The natural result is lowered metabolic rates, cravings and binging. Most binges would probably never occur if dieting were replaced with better food choices which would promote a slow, steady drop in weight, rather than an overly rapid weight loss.

Skipped meals and skimpy portions are not effective for permanent weight control and are not a part of this program.

An Optimal Weight-loss Menu

Now that you know what not to do, let's build a program that takes pounds off and keeps them off. The basis of this program is a way of eating that promotes weight control naturally, without counting calories and without skimpy portions.

Let's first look at *carbohydrates*. The starchy white inside of a potato is mostly complex carbohydrate, which is simply a chemist's term for molecules made up of many natural sugars linked together. When you eat a potato, that carbohydrate is gradually broken apart into simple sugars, which are absorbed and used by the body. Rice, wheat, oats, and other grains are rich in complex carbohydrates, as are beans and nearly all vegetables.

In the past, many people believed that starchy foods were fattening. They would avoid carbohydrate-rich potatoes, rice, bread, and pasta. People would take a baked potato, which has only 95 calories, and top it with a pat or two of butter, and sometimes add sour cream, grated cheese, or bacon bits. As they gained weight, they blamed the potato. But we now know that what was fattening was not the potato, but the greasy toppings that were added to it.

✦ Carbohydrate-rich foods are actually low in calories.
✦ A gram of carbohydrate (about ¹/₃₀ ounce) = 4 calories.

That is why a slice of bread has only 70 calories and an ear of corn only 120. A chicken breast, which contains no carbohydrate, has fully 386 calories. In contrast, starchy foods are low-calorie foods.

Compare that to fatty foods. A gram of fat has nine calories, more than twice the calorie content of carbohydrate. It is only when carbohydrate-rich foods are covered with fatty toppings that lots of calories are added.

Look at how this works with actual foods: You are planning a candlelight dinner for two. A nice spaghetti dinner with some fresh vegetables, perhaps a glass of wine. A one-cup serving of spaghetti topped with $1/2$ cup of tomato sauce has about 200 calories. But if we decided to add ground beef to the sauce, look what happens: the spaghetti dinner suddenly has 365 calories. The fat in ground beef holds a lot of calories.

Let's take another example: A half-cup serving of mashed potatoes has 70 calories. A tablespoon of butter on top adds fully 108 calories. In the process a low-calorie food becomes a high-calorie food. In other words, fatty toppings are high in calories, but the carbohydrate-rich potatoes, spaghetti, bread, etc., are not.

Food and Fatty Toppings

Potato (1 med.) = 95 calories

Potato (1 med.) + Butter (1 Tbs) = 203 calories

Potato (1 med.) + Butter (1 Tbs) + Cheese (1 oz) = 317 calories

---

There may be an advantage to whole unprocessed grains, such as rice, cereal, or corn, as opposed to grain which has been ground up into flour (e.g. bread or pasta). Some evidence shows that we tend to extract more calories from the ground-up varieties, perhaps because the process of "digestion" has been begun for us.

There are other important virtues of carbohydrates. They cannot add *directly* to your fat stores. We do not have any "carbohydrate storage areas" on our bellies or thighs. If the body is to store the energy of carbohydrates in fat, it has to chemically convert the carbohydrate molecules into fat. This process consumes a fair number of calories. As a result:

✦

*Calories from carbohydrates
are not as likely to increase body fat
as are the same number of calories from fats.*

✦

In addition, *carbohydrates boost your metabolism.* Plant-based meals tend to increase the metabolic rate slightly. Here is how it works: Carbohydrate breaks down in the body to various sugars. Sugars cause insulin to be released which, in turn, leads to the production of two natural hormones, norepinephrine and thryoid hormone (T 3). T 3 and norepi-nephrine both increase the metabolic rate. The result is more effective calorie burning.

Carbohydrates Increase Metabolism

Carbohydrates → Sugar → Insulin

Norepinephrine & T3

Increased Metabolism
(More effective calorie burning)

So starchy foods are naturally low in calories, they cannot be automatically added to body fat, and they help boost your metabolic rate so that calories are burned off a bit faster.

✦ Carbohydrate-rich vegetables, beans, and grains are the best friends of anyone trying to shed some pounds.

Now here is a critical point:

✦ Complex carbohydrates are found only in plants.

Grains, such as bread, spaghetti, and rice are loaded with carbohydrates. Beans and vegetables are also high in carbohydrates. But there are virtually no complex carbohydrates in chicken, fish, beef, pork, eggs, or dairy products. The more animal products you eat, the more you are pushing carbohydrate-rich vegetable foods off your plate. That is one reason why the most effective weight-control programs use vegetarian menus.

There is an added bonus to foods from plants: fiber. Grains, beans, and vegetables contain fiber, which adds texture and makes them filling and satisfying. Fiber is what people used to call roughage, the part of plants that resists digestion in the small intestine. The value of fiber was not appreciated until relatively recently, and so it was often removed by refining methods. The result was white bread instead of whole-grain breads, white rice instead of brown rice, and baked goods that were more densely packed with calories and less satisfying than they would have been had the fiber been left in. Fiber adds a hearty texture to foods but has virtually no calories.

Like complex carbohydrates, fiber is found only in plants. Grains, such as wheat, oats, rye, corn, rice, and the breads, cereals, and other foods that are made from them are loaded with fiber. Vegetables of all kinds and legumes, such as beans, peas, and lentils, are also rich in fiber.

Animal products contain no fiber at all. To the extent that animal products are added to the diet, the fiber content is reduced. Americans now consume only 10-20 grams of fiber per day, on average, which is about half of what we should have. The reason, of course, is the penchant for animal products and refined plant foods, which unfortunately displace the fiber-rich foods. *But do not feel that you must calculate your fiber intake.* When you center your diet on high-carbohydrate foods, such as whole grains, beans, and vegetables, the fiber content of your diet will increase naturally. As you will see in Part II, the result will be meals that are satisfying and filling. When we discuss the value of carbohydrate-rich foods and fiber, you can simplify this by thinking in terms of foods from plants versus animal products. A plant-based diet is rich in carbohydrate and fiber. Animal products are devoid of them. The result is that plant-based diets promote slimness, while Animal products promote overweight.

Charlene:
Beating a Weight Problem

Charlene wanted to lose 30 pounds. In fact, she had wanted to lose these same 30 pounds for several years. She had tried several different diets, including some with formula drinks, and had also tried diet pills. None of these were effective over the long run, although all had seemed to help temporarily. When I met her, she was avoiding all carbohydrates. She skipped breakfast, had yogurt and turkey slices for lunch, and usually ate frozen dietetic meals for dinner. Her weight had been essentially the same for months.

I suggested that, instead of avoiding starchy foods, she make them the center of her diet. Breakfast was to be hot cereal and fruit. At work, she could make lunch from dried soups. For dinner, she was to make a pot of rice, as much as she could eat, or, if she preferred, she could have potatoes or other starchy foods instead. She was also to include vegetables and beans or lentils at dinner. Because this "diet" included a rather large quantity of food, she worried that she might actually gain weight on it. But some rather simple calculations showed that the calorie content of this menu was actually very modest. She lost weight very gradually, but about 10 months later, the 30 extra pounds were gone.

The Negative Calorie Effect

Many people still believe that the number of calories in any given food tells you just how fattening that food is likely to be. For example, a cup of rice has about 220 calories. Three slices of bologna also have 220 calories. So some people assume that these two foods have exactly the same effect on the waistline.

They don't. The very same number of calories coming from bologna and from rice have very different effects. The bologna tends to be fattening, as a general rule, while the rice does not.

Rice does provide calories to run the body's functions. And theoretically it is possible for unused calories from rice to be stored as fat. But it turns out that rice is much less fattening than the same number of calories from bologna, other meats, or other fatty foods. Rice—like other carbohydrate-rich foods—has a way of naturally *reducing* the calories that are available for fat storage.

You might think of this as a "negative calorie effect." One of the most exciting concepts in the science of weight control in many years is the fact that certain foods can actually assist in the *loss* of fat.

By now, it will come as no surprise to you that carbohydrate-rich foods are power foods for weight control. But let's see what the "negative calorie effect" really means. Then, we'll look at 20 foods that encourage this effect and which you can eat freely. In reality there are far more than 20, and by the time you are done with this book, I hope you will have gone far beyond the old-fashioned notion of counting calories and limiting portion size. The key is not how much you eat, but, instead, the types of foods you eat.

When you think of carbohydrate, think, for example, of rice. A rice grain is a seed, designed by nature to start a new rice plant. The starchy white interior of a rice grain consists mainly of complex carbohydrates that nourish the seed as it sprouts and grows. The same is true of beans, potatoes, apples, and many other plants. The starchy carbohydrate interior provides nourishment for the tiny growing plant.

For millions of years, humans and other primates have plucked fruits from trees and roots from the ground and have taken advantage of carbohydrate's capacity to nourish us. What is remarkable is that these foods provide energy with relatively little tendency to cause overweight. In many Asian countries, for example, where rice is still the center of the diet and huge amounts of rice are consumed, people tend to remain slim.

While carbohydrates provide calories for the body, they also have ways of counteracting the storage of some of these calories as fat, and also encourage the burning of stored calories:

First, as we saw earlier, a substantial number of the calories in carbohydrates are used up as carbohydrates are turned to fat. Let me give you some numbers: For every 100 calories of carbohydrate that your body tries to store as fat, 23 are lost in the process of breaking down carbohydrate molecules and building fat molecules from them. That means that, of the 220 calories in a cup of rice, about 50 calories are used up just in the chemical processing. Leaving grains whole, like rice, cereals, or corn, rather than grinding them into flour to make bread or pasta, also causes them to release fewer calories.

But that is just the beginning. In addition, because carbohydrate increases the body's metabolism, more calories are burned off as the metabolism increases. The metabolism-boosting effect causes more of the calories in *all the foods you eat* to be burned. When that happens, they cannot be turned into fat.

It is similar to the effect of turning up a car's idle. More gas is used up; there is less in the tank, less to spill on the ground, and less to use in the future, because it has been burned.

Another part of the "negative calorie effect" of carbohydrates is that they are the part of the diet that tells the body when it has had enough food. Your body does not just pay attention to how much you have eaten. It actually has a way to monitor how much carbohydrate is coming in. When it has had enough, it reduces the feeling of hunger. Carbohydrates are the cue the body needs. So, if there is a lot of carbohydrate on your plate, you will tend to eat to feel satisfied and to turn down the drive to fill your plate. The natural sugar in fruits, called fructose, also has an appetite-reducing effect.

What this means is that if you have included generous amounts of rice, potatoes, beans, fruits, and other carbohydrate-rich foods on your meals, the calories in pork chops, salad oil, and other fattening foods are less likely to find their way onto your fork.

How do you get these "negative calorie effects?" You will not get them from steak or fried chicken, because there is virtually no complex carbohydrate in fish, chicken, beef, milk, eggs, or any other animal product. Complex carbohydrates are found only in plants. Grains, vegetables, and beans are loaded with them. That is why vegetarian foods are such powerful foods for permanent weight control.

If you like, you can forget technical terms like carbohydrate. As long as your diet is made from grains, beans, vegetables, and fruits, rather than animal products, it will be naturally rich in carbohydrate.

20 Foods You Can Eat
in Virtually Unlimited Portions

Listed below are 20 foods that you should feel free to eat in very generaous portions. Unless you are really stuffing yourself, you can eat as much of these as you want. In fact, there are many more than 20, as you have learned. One caveat: Enjoy these with no butter, margarine or oily toppings—fats are fattening!

Corn	Celery
Rice	Peas
Potatoes	Cauliflower
Lettuce (all varieties)	Tomatoes
Broccoli	Cabbage
Carrots	Oranges
Black beans	Apples
Kidney beans	Grapefruit
Spinach	Bananas

Cutting Out Fats and Oils

Now for the most important part of the food prescription:

+ Cut out the fats and oils.
+ Fats and oils are packed with calories.
+ Fat in foods is fat on you.

These are the most calorie-dense part of the foods we eat. As we noted previously, every single gram of fat or oil holds nine calories. This is true for all fats and oils: beef fat, chicken fat, fish oil, vegetable oil, and any other kind of fat or oil.

In the May 1991 issue of the *American Journal of Clinical Nutrition*, researchers at Cornell University published the results of a fascinating experiment. They had kept volunteers on different diets for several weeks. They found that those who ate foods that were very low in fat and high in carbohydrates lost weight steadily, *without limiting how much they ate*. But those on high-fat diets could not effectively lose weight even if they ate skimpy portions. A similar phenomenon was found by Dr. T. Colin Campbell of the China Health Study, a massive and on-going research undertaking.[2] His team found that Chinese populations eat a very high carbohydrate diet with enormous quantities of rice. They eat very little in the way of animal products, and so, get little fat in their diets. Overall, their diets contain more calories than most Americans eat, but they stay much slimmer, both because of the very low fat content and high carbohydrate content of the diet, and because they stay physically active, which we will discuss later. The first key to emphasize is the need to shift from fatty foods to carbohydrates.

There are various kinds of fat. The main categories discussed by dietitians are *saturated fat*, which is common in animal products and is solid at room temperature, and *unsaturated fat*, which is common in vegetable oils and is liquid at room temperature. Different kinds of fat have different effects on your cholesterol level. But:

✦ For weight control, we need to be concerned about
all forms of fat.
✦ All fats and oils have the same calorie content:
9 calories in every gram.

About 40 percent of the calories most Americans get every day come from fat. For a typical 2000-calorie menu, that is 800 calories each day just from fats and oils in our foods. By cutting out most of the fats in our diet, we can cut out hundreds of calories. To put it another way, if all the foods we eat are very low in fat, we can eat far more food than we could on a high-fat diet, without more calories.

We should cut our fat intake from 40 percent of the calories we eat down to about 15 percent. Eating 15 percent of our calories from fat is a substantial reduction. It is a powerful weight-reducing step and yields other tremendous benefits as well. We must go on a "search and destroy" mission for fat. *Be on the look-out for fat in the two forms in which it comes: animal fat and vegetable oil.*

Look out for ALL fats!

Animal fat was designed by nature to act as a calorie-storage area for animals. When you eat animal fat, you are eating all those stored calories. Animal fat is not only on the outside of a cut of meat. It is marbled through the lean part, too, almost like a sponge holding water. So, if you are eating meat you are eating someone else's fat and someone else's concentrated stored calories. It will put fat on you. Let's take some examples:

Imagine that we are making tacos. Let's compare two recipes for taco filling, one made with ground beef and the other with beans. Beef is high in fat; three ounces of ground beef hold about 225 calories. Beans are very low in fat, and three ounces hold only about 80 calories. So we can cut out nearly two-thirds of the calorie content by switching from the beef recipe to the bean recipe. A big part of the difference is the very high fat content of the ground beef and the very low fat content of beans. About 60 percent of the calories in ground

Food	Percentage calories from fat
Potato	less than 1 %
Peas	3 %
Black beans	4 %
Macaroni noodles	4 %
Vegetarian baked beans	4 %
Rice	less than 5 %
Cauliflower	6 %
Spinach	7 %
Broccoli	8 %
Wheat bread	15 %
Whole milk	49 %
2% milk	35 %
Extra lean gound beef	54 %
Ground beef	60 %

beef come from fat. This is a huge load of calories that do nothing good for the body and do a lot of harm, from promoting heart disease to increasing cancer risk, and, of course, fattening you up.

Take a look at the fat content of various foods in the chart on the previous page. Remember, the fat contents listed here are percentages of calories, not percentages by weight. This is a critical difference. Whole milk, for example, is 3.3 percent fat

Whole Milk

3.3% Fat By Weight

49% Fat By Percent of Calories

2% Milk

2% Fat By Weight

35% Fat By Percent of Calories

by weight, because it is loaded with water. But 49 percent of its calories come from fat. Milk that is two percent fat by weight is actually about 35 percent fat as a percentage of calories. It is actually not a low-fat product at all.

"Extra lean" ground beef is really not so lean either: it derives 54 percent of its calories from fat. It is an abysmal food for people concerned about their waistlines. Even McDonald's McLean DeLuxe burger is not a low-fat food. Although the company advertises it as "91 percent fat-free," they are using the weight percentage, not the calorie percentage. By calories, the McLean DeLuxe patty is 49 percent fat, hardly something anyone would recommend.

By calorie content, here's a listing of common meat cuts:

Common Meat Cuts	
Cut	Percentage of calories from fat
Chuck roast	51 %
Rib eye steak	63 %
Short loin porterhouse	64 %
Hotdogs	82 %
Bologna	83 %
Most beans, grains, vegetables	less than 10 %

Even the beef industry in its "lean" advertisments of the "skinniest six" beef specimens could not find any cuts of meat that are anywhere near the fat content of beans, grains, or vegetables:

"Skinniest Six" Meat Cuts	
Cut	Percentage of calories from fat
Tenderloin	41 %
Top loin	40 %
Sirloin	38 %
Round tip	36 %
Eye of round	32 %
Top round	29 %
Most beans, grains, vegetables	less than 10 %

All of these have many times the fat content of typical vegetables, beans, grains, and fruits.

The problem with meats, including poultry and fish, is that they are muscles, and muscles are made up of protein and fat. They contain no fiber at all and virtually no carbohydrate.

Advertisers sometimes claim that chicken and fish are low-fat foods. Are they? Let's look at the worst and the best of the poultry line:

Poultry	Percentage of calories from fat
Chicken frank	68 %
Roasted chicken	51 %
White meat w/out skin	23 %
Most beans, grains, vegetables	less than 10 %

The chicken also contributes about 85 mg. of cholesterol. In addition, chicken pushes carbohydrates and fiber off your plate. No matter how chicken is prepared, it cannot get its calorie level down to that of the truly healthful foods, because chicken, like all meats, is permeated by fat and contains no complex carbohydrates or fiber. *Fat always has more calories than carbohydrate.*

Some people eat fish in the hope that fish oil will reduce their cholesterol levels. Actually, fish oils reduce triglycerides but do not reduce cholesterol levels. And it should be remembered that fish oils are as fattening as any other oils or fats. Like all fats and oils, they contain nine calories per gram.

Different types of fish differ greatly in their fat content:

Fish	Percentage of calories from fat
Chinook salmon	52 %
Atlantic salmon	40 %
Swordfish	30 %
Halibut	19 %
Snapper	12 %
Sole	9 %
Haddock	8 %

Many of these are as bad as other animal products. Others are in the same ballpark as vegetables as far as their fat content goes, but this does not make them recommended foods. Remember fish contains no complex carbohydrates and no fiber, and tends to displace these foods from the meal. All fish products also contain cholesterol and far too much protein, (see pages 41-44) in addition to contamination problems. So, fish is still not a health food, although certain types of fish are much lower in fat than are beef and poultry.

In summary, meats, poultry, and fish have two main problems for those concerned about their weight:

First, like all muscles, they have inherent fat, adding concentrated calories.

Second, because muscle tissues are mainly just protein and fat, they reduce the carbohydrate and fiber content of the diet. They displace the fiber and carbohydrates that are essential to a satisfying and metabolism-boosting menu.

✦

The first prescription for cutting the fat is the V-word:
vegetarian foods are power foods
for weight control.

The second issue is vegetable oil.

✦

Vegetable oils have received a good reputation because they contain no cholesterol and are low in saturated fats. But their calorie content is the same as any other kind of fat. That should be emphasized. *All fats and all oils, regardless of type (lard, pork fat, chicken fat, olive oil, fish oil, etc.), are packed with calories: nine calories per gram.* They are all the enemies of those in search of a slimmer waistline.

Let's take an example with vegetable oils: As you know, a potato is a low-fat food that is also modest in calories. Only about one percent of the calories in a potato come from fat.

When the potato is baked or prepared as mashed potatoes, no extra oil is added. But if the potato is cut into french fries and dropped in cooking oil, its fat content soars up to 40 percent or more. As a result, its calorie content doubles or even triples.

Compare the fat content of a doughnut (50 %), which is fried in oil, to a bagel (8 %), which is not. The doughnut has more than six times the fat of the bagel.

Fat in foods adds easily to your fat stores.

1 Large Raw Potato		2 Regular Fries
70 Calories	Frying	440 Calories
.1 gram fat		23 grams fat

Little or no conversion is needed in the body before the fat we eat passes through the digestive tract and the blood stream to the fat tissues of the body. But the energy in carbohydrates cannot be easily stored as fat. The body has to do a considerable amount of work before those calories can be stored, and many calories are lost in the process.

Fats Are Calorie-Dense	
Carbohydrate	4 calories per gram
Protein	4 calories per gram
Fat	**9 calories per gram**

There are other serious problems with fats, too. Fat in foods contributes substantially to the risk of several forms of cancer (breast, colon, prostate, and others), heart disease, diabetes, gallstones, and numerous other problems as well. Although animal fats are the worst, vegetable oils also increase health problems.

A low-fat menu is a recipe for a slim, healthy body. It can take some getting used to because, unfortunately, people crave high-fat foods. Grease is like an addicting substance. We all have a tendency to return to fried chicken, greasy burgers, potato chips, and fried onion rings, so be on the look-out. It is easier to cut them out entirely than to continually tease oneself with occasional greasy foods.

Getting Free from the Fat in Foods

As you know from the above discussion, shifting away from fat and toward high-fiber foods means getting away from animal products. Cutting out animal products can greatly reduce your fat consumption. Avoiding added vegetable oils and fried foods is another very powerful step. Here are some suggestions on how to do it:

Salad Dressings: Salad dressings can be packed with fat. A salad made of one cup of romaine lettuce with half a tomato holds only 20 calories. But look what adding a tablespoon of dressing will do:

Salad dressing (1 Tbsp.)	Fat content
Catalina french dressing	5.5 grams of fat (65 calories)
vinegar and oil (50/50 mix)	8 grams of fat (72 calories)
Good Seasons Zesty Italian	9.2 grams of fat (85 calories)

So the salad with dressing has four to five times the calories of a salad without dressing.

Low-fat or no-fat dressings cut down substantially on the fat content. Look at the brands that are now available at the grocery store, often in the "dietetic section." Or you might prefer a sprinkle of lemon or lime juice as a dressing for salad or vegetables. A tablespoon of lemon or lime juice has no fat and only four calories. You may also find that you enjoy the taste of fresh spinach, chick peas, tomatoes, or other salad ingredients with no dressing at all.

Baked Goods: In recent years, nutritionists have made distinctions between saturated (animal fat, tropical, and hydro-genated oils) and unsaturated (most vegetable) oils, because the former contribute to heart problems. But if our goal is to slim down, the issue is much simpler: all kinds of fats and oils are problems. They are all packed with calories. Some baked goods, such as bagels, pretzels, and many breads, are usually quite low in fat. On the other hand, croissants, cakes, pies, and cookies tend to be very high in fat. Commercially packaged goods list their ingredients on the label. The ingredients are listed in decreasing order of their quantities, so if oil is one of the first ingredients, there is probably more of it than if it is one of the last listed ingredients. In addition, most labels provide enough information to allow you to calculate the actual fat content, using the simple formula on the next page (page36).

We do need some fat in the diet. But we need only a fraction of what most of us typically get. A small amount of fat is inherent in grains, legumes, and vegetables. This is all the body needs. Children can (and perhaps should) have a bit more fat in their diet. Breast milk is naturally higher in fat for the needs of growing infants. The natural process of weaning eliminates this nutrient when it is no longer appropriate.

How To Check The Fat Content Of Foods

How much fat is in foods we eat?

What is important is the percentage of calories that comes from fat. (The percentage of fat by weight is not important, because it can be easily thrown off by the water content of products.)

Some manufacturers are starting to list the percentage figure, but, if they do not, it is still easy to calculate. On the information panel on the package, notice the number of grams of fat in one serving. Multiply by nine (every gram of fat contains nine calories). Then divide by the number of calories per serving. Then multiply by 100.

$$\frac{\text{grams of fat} \times 9}{\text{calories in serving}} \times 100 = \% \text{ calories from fat}$$

Let's try an example. Here is an information label from a supposedly low-calorie pizza:

NUTRITIONAL INFORMATION

Serving size ... 1.0 oz	Carbohydrates ... 7.2 g
Servings per pkg ... 8	Fat ... 2.5 g
Calories ... 65	Sodium ... 74 mg
Protein ... 3.1 g	Cholesterol ... 1 mg

This serving is incredibly small, so all the numbers will be artificially low. But even so, the key to look for is the percentage of calories that come from fat. One serving contains 2.5 grams of fat. If we multiply by nine and divide by the number of calories per serving (65), we come out with .35. Then multiplying by 100 gives us 35 percent. This means that 35 percent of the calories in this product are from fat. This is better than fried chicken or a hot dog, but still higher than we want. Not such a healthful entree after all.

$$\frac{2.5 \times 9}{65} = .35 \times 100 = 35\% \text{ of calories from fat}$$

Reggie:
Swearing Off Grease

Reggie called himself a 'grease addict.' Potato chips, French fries, buttered popcorn, peanuts, peanut butter, and onion rings were all part of his routine. He had been fairly slim until he reached about 25 when his waistline gradually began to expand. Now, at 40, he is about 20 pounds overweight. His daily intake of fatty foods had a predictable effect.

He did not plan to give up any foods totally. But as an experiment, he decided that for three weeks he would eat only low-fat vegetarian meals. From a set of recipes, he made bean entrees with lots of vegetables on the side. There was no limit on amounts, but he was very strict to omit all oils, margarine, salad dressings, and all meats and dairy products. After three weeks, he had lost about three pounds. That was not a big drop, but he found that he had lost all desire for greasy foods, and now associated them with his weight problems. So he decided to stick with his new way of eating for three more weeks. He lost five more pounds. A month later, he had lost another 5 pounds. He now weighs the same as he did in college.

His friend Morris adopted the same program. He weighed 275 pounds when he started. Without limiting calories, he lost 80 pounds. His girlfriend used the same method to drop from 150 to 120 pounds.

Chemical fat substitutes have recently emerged in the news. *Simplesse*, made by the NutraSweet Company, is made of a protein that simulates the texture of grease on the tongue. Because it changes consistency when heated, Simplesse can only be used in foods which are not baked or fried. *Olestra* is a sucrose polyester made by Procter and Gamble. It is designed to taste and feel like fat, but is indigestible and unabsorbable. Its safety is a matter of vigorous dispute; some contend that Olestra causes cancer and liver problems.

I find it impossible to be enthusiastic about these products. Like chemical sweeteners, their safety remains in doubt. In addition, they reinforce the taste for fat, rather than helping you to get away from the taste for grease.

To reduce the fat content of the diet, low-fat vegetarian foods are ideal. Vegetarian foods are obviously free of the animal fat that permeates meats, poultry, and fish. Steering clear of fried foods and added oils is the other half of the equation. Spaghetti with tomato sauce, bean burritos, vegetable curries, baked potatoes, and salads are a few examples of foods that can be very low in fat, yet delicious.

Check Your Knowledge

Let's review. For each pair below, see if you can pick which is lower in fat. You'll find the answers below. Do not skip this part. It is easy, but important.

Which is lower in fat?
1. Fried chicken vs. broiled top round beef
2. Leanest beef vs. leanest chicken
3. Leanest chicken vs. vegetarian baked beans
4. Leanest beef vs. rice
5. Leanest chicken vs. potato
6. Spaghetti with tomato sauce vs. a Lean Cuisine spaghetti with meatballs dinner
7. Spaghetti with meat sauce vs. spaghetti with tomato sauce
8. Fast-food meat taco vs. fast-food bean burrito
9. Cheddar cheese vs. bread
10. Peanut butter vs. rice
11. Ice cream vs. jelly beans
12. Baked potato vs. french fries
13. Doughnut vs. bagel

Answers
(The numbers given are percentages of calories from fat):
1. Broiled top round beef (38 %) is lower in fat than fried chicken (50 % fat), but both are high-fat foods.
2. The leanest chicken is about 20 % fat, and lower than the leanest beef (29 % fat), although both are high in fat compared to grains, beans, vegetables, and fruits.
3. Vegetarian baked beans (4 % fat) are much lower in fat than even the very leanest chicken (20 %).
4. Rice (0.8 %) is much lower in fat than the leanest beef (29 % fat).
5. A potato (1 %) is much lower in fat than the leanest chicken (20 % fat).

6. Spaghetti with tomato sauce (6 %) is much lower in fat than a Lean Cuisine spaghetti with meatballs dinner (23 %).
7. Spaghetti with tomato sauce (6 %) is lower in fat than spaghetti with meat sauce (35 %).
8. A fast-food bean burrito (31 %) is lower in fat than a fast-food meat taco (50 %). A home-made burrito can be much lower in fat.
9. Bread (16 %) is much lower in fat than cheddar cheese (74 %). Most cheeses are extremely high in fat.
10. Rice (0.8 %) is much lower in fat than peanut butter (78 %).
11. Jelly beans (0.8 %) are much lower in fat than ice cream (48 %), although both hold a very large amount of sugar.
12. A baked potato (1 %) is much lower in fat than french fries (47 %).
13. A bagel (8 %) is much lower in fat than a doughnut (50 %).

Carbohydrate-rich foods are vital for long-term weight control. Take the carbohydrate test below:

Which has more carbohydrate?
1. A fish fillet vs. broccoli
2. Bread vs. beef
3. Milk vs. potato
4. Cheese vs. rice

Answers:
(The numbers given are percentages of calories from carbohydrate):
1. Broccoli is 78 % carbohydrate. A fish fillet has no carbohydrate at all.
2. Bread is 75 % carbohydrate. Beef has no carbohydrate at all.
3. A potato is 93 % carbohydrate. Milk is 30 % carbohydrate, in the form of simple sugar.
4. Rice has much more carbohydrate (89 %) than cheese (1 %).

What About Protein?

Protein is the subject of many myths. The bottom line on protein is this: High-protein diets are dangerous. Many formula diets emphasize high-protein foods and contain very little carbohydrate. This type of diet is not a formula for success. It can cause a rapid, and usually temporary, water loss. But usually the weight comes back on very quickly.

In addition, there are serious dangers to high-protein diets: osteoporosis and kidney disease. The bone-thinning disease of osteoporosis is an epidemic in the U.S., and protein has apparently been a big part of the cause. High-protein diets cause calcium to be lost in the urine. This has been shown repeatedly in scientific studies. When subjects consume foods that are overly high in protein, especially animal protein, they excrete calcium. For example, if volunteers were to eat meals with a substantial meat content and later have their urine tested, calcium would often be found in the urine. Since Americans tend to eat meat daily, it is likely that they are routinely excreting calcium. The calcium does not come from the meat. It comes from their bones.

There are several theories that scientists have used to explain this. The amino acids which make up protein and are released when protein is digested make the blood slightly acidic. In the process of buffering this acid, calcium is pulled from the bones. Ultimately it is discarded in the urine. In addition, meat protein is very high in what are called "sulfur-containing amino acids." These are suspected of being particularly likely to leach calcium from the bones.

While many of us grew up being taught to make sure we got enough protein, the fact is we have gotten too much. Our bodies only need a fraction of what we generally get. When we eat two or three times the amount of protein the body can use, much of it is broken down and excreted. In the process, it not only interferes with the calcium balance of the body, it can also overwork the kidneys. The excess of amino acids acts as a diuretic, increasing the flow of urine. The amino acids eventually break down to urea, which acts as a diuretic, too. The overall effect is to force the kidneys to work much harder than they should. The nephrons, which are the kidneys' filter units, gradually die off in the process.

We need protein in the diet, but we do not need a large overdose of protein. The problems of calcium loss and kidney damage occur, not just in those who consume high-protein formulas, but in people who consume meat, chicken, or fish on a regular basis.

The best advice about protein is to stick with plant sources. A varied menu of grains, beans, and vegetables contains more than enough protein for human needs. There is no need to carefully combine proteins. Any variety of plant foods provides sufficient protein. When meats are included, the protein content easily becomes more than the body can handle safely. For example, if you were to have a single seven-ounce serving of roast beef, you would get 62 grams of protein. This one serving contains more than the recommended daily allowance of protein for a whole day (a range of 44-56 gms., depending on your age and level of activity), unless you are pregnant or nursing.

Let's take a look at two other high-protein products, egg

whites and skim milk. Doctors learned long ago that egg yolks were loaded with cholesterol. A single egg yolk contains 213 mg. of cholesterol (and is 80 % fat). That is even more cholesterol than in an eight-ounce steak. But while many doctors now recommend avoiding egg yolks, some still encourage the consumption of egg whites because they contain protein. Well, the fact is that egg whites contain *too much* protein. Of the calories in an egg white, fully 85 % are from protein. That is a huge amount that no one needs. (In addition, salmonella bacteria are an increasing problem in eggs, even those with intact shells.)

Protein Myths

1. Milk for strong bones
2. Egg whites are good
3. Vegetarians do not get enough protein.

Skim milk is a similar wrong turn. Because of the high saturated fat content of whole milk, many people have chosen skim dairy products. Getting rid of the dairy fat is certainly a good idea, because the fat in whole milk, butter, cheese, cream, and ice cream will tend to increase cholesterol levels and elevate cancer risk. But after the fat is removed, skim milk is hardly a health food. It contains no fiber, and no complex carbohydrates, but has a substantial amount of lactose sugar (55 % of calories). Antibiotics are also frequently present in milk products, due to their routine use on farms.

If you thought you needed milk for strong bones, you have been the victim of an extremely aggressive advertising program by the dairy industry which was not based on good science. The fact is that people in countries which consume milk routinely tend to have weaker bones than those in countries which avoid milk. Osteoporosis is more likely due to excess protein in the diet and to sedentary living. It is not due to a "milk deficiency," and milk consumption does not slow the osteoprosis that commonly occurs in older women.

There are also concerns about the *type* of protein in milk. Milk proteins often cause allergies and other health problems. There are indications that milk proteins contribute to juvenile-onset diabetes, and specialized cow proteins (antibodies) are now known to cause colic in infants. Like it or not, nature designed cow's milk for baby cows, not for people.

Limit Alcohol

In general, health recommendations have been mixed on alcohol: Modest alcohol consumption—one to two drinks per day—does not promote heart problems. On the other hand, even small amounts of alcohol increase the risk of breast cancer and contribute to birth defects. And, of course, beyond modest use, alcohol contributes to many other very serious health problems, from accidents to heart disease, cancer, neurological disorders, and digestive problems.

What about its effect on your waistline? This is no mystery. Alcohol is fattening. People who consume beer, wine, or mixed drinks on a regular basis get a big load of extra calories, as this list shows:

Drink	Calories
Wine (4 oz.)	85
Light Beer (12 oz.)	100
Beer (12 oz.)	150
Liquor (1.5 oz.)	124
100 proof gin, rum, vodka or whiskey	

These figures are not presented for you to remember, but rather to illustrate that the alcohol in these beverages packs a significant number of calories.

What is important about alcohol, however, is not just its calorie content. The important point is this: *Alcohol adds to the calories you are already consuming, rather than displacing any.* For example, if you were to eat four bread sticks before dinner, you would eat a bit less at dinner. The 150 calories in the bread would displace about the same amount from the food you would have later. But alcohol does not seem to have this same sort of compensatory mechanism.[3] If you substitute a beer for the bread sticks, it also holds 150 calories, and the calories from alcohol are not compensated for by eating less later. The calories in alcohol *add* to what you eat.

The presumption is that although soft drinks hold about the same number of calories as beer (a can of cola holds about 155 calories), they are much more likely to be compensated for later than are the calories in alcoholic beverages, since the calories in soft drinks come from sugar. For mixed drinks, the calories in the drink mix are not so likely to contribute to your girth as the calories in the alcohol which is added to it. This is not a recommendation for colas and drink mixes. The point is that alcohol can really widen your waistline. For alcoholics, the effects are different. Alcoholics often consume less food than do non-alcoholics and are deficient in a host of nutrients.

Sweets and Sweeteners

Concentrated sugars, such as hard candies, are just chunks of simple sugars and lack any fiber or water. As a result, they are as concentrated a form of calories as can be found in a carbohydrate food. If you consume large quantities of sugary foods, such as sweets and sodas, you will get more calories than the body needs.

But even so, sugars are not nearly as calorie-dense as fats. If you are not controlling the amount of fat you are eating, there is little point in worrying about sugar.

Often, sugar is not the main problem in sweets. In cookies, pies, and cakes, there may be a lot of sugar, but there is usually a huge amount of fat, too.

Sweets	Percentage of calories from fat
Haagen-Dazs ice cream	57 %
Hershey dark chocolate bar	50 %
Chips Ahoy cookies	42 %
Pillsbury German Chocolate cake	40 %

When selecting sweet foods, pick those with the lowest amount of fat. How about fruit for dessert? And sodas should be replaced with spritzers or water.

Forget artificial sweeteners. They are no answer to weight problems. First of all, they do not seem to have much power to help in weight control. Using an artificial sweetener instead of a teaspoon of sugar saves you only 16 calories. But just two grams of fat hold more calories than the teaspoon of sugar. That is not to say that you should consume sugar, but it is to say that artificial sweeteners are a distraction from the real dietary issues, which for most people relate to the fat content of the diet.

More importantly, artificial sweeteners are poisonous. We have seen this over and over again. Cyclamates can cause cancer. The same may be true of saccharin, although it remains on the market with warning labels on each package. Aspartame, marketed under the name NutraSweet, has problems of its own. Substantial evidence links aspartame to a variety of effects on the brain. Headaches are common, and there is currently a scientific debate over whether aspartame can cause grand mal seizures and whether children, including babies developing in the womb, may suffer brain damage if exposed to aspartame. I see no value in chemical sweeteners.

Check Your Knowledge

Try each question. Do not skip any. Answers are listed below.

1. How do alcoholic beverages affect weight problems?
2. What problems are caused by diets with too much protein?
3. Is there a lot of fat in pies and cookies?
4. True or false: As far as protein is concerned, the more the better.
5. True or false: Vegetarians get enough protein without carefully combining foods.

Answers:

1. Alcohol contains calories, and we do not compensate for this by eating less later.
2. Osteoporosis and kidney problems.
3. Yes.
4. False. We need some protein, and the amount in plant foods is sufficient. Adding high-protein products is not healthful.
5. True.

Watch Out For Stuffing

Most overweight people do not overeat. Most actually eat less than thin people do. But some people do overeat. For one of many reasons, they are "stuffers;" they keep eating long after others would have had enough. It is important to identify whether you are a member of that minority of overweight people who do tend to overeat so you can learn what to do about it. Let's look at three principal reasons for overeating:

1. *The Restrained-Eater Phenomenon:* As we saw earlier, one big reason for an episode of overeating is the re- strained-eater phenomenon, which kicks in after periods of very-low-calorie dieting. This can affect anyone, even people who have never had a tendency to binge or to overeat for any psychological reason. The key, of course, is to avoid the very- low-calorie regimens that tend to produce binges.

2. *Eating in Response to Emotions:* Ask yourself these questions:

✦ Is food your usual answer to stress?
✦ Do you eat when you are not at all hungry?
✦ Do you eat throughout the day?

If the answer to any of these is yes, then this section may be for you.

Some people eat when they are under stress. Depres- sion, anxiety, hurt feelings, anger, or sadness are answered with a trip to the kitchen. This is easy to identify, and a bit harder to remedy. Do not expect to plumb the depths of your psyche and rearrange its contents in short order. For now, you need to make a plan to compensate for this tendency.

Anticipate that from time to time, like it or not, you will become angry or sad or frustrated with things, and plan to deal with these feelings in another way. Is there someone you can talk to, or someone you can call? If food is serving as a comfort, what other comforts can you take advantage of? For example, are there certain places, photographs, books, or clothes that serve as comforts, too?

Deal with emotions in ways that are inconsistent with eating. For example, if you plan to get together with a friend, be with someone who is not preoccupied with eating, and pick a place where eating will not occur—meet in a park or office instead of a restaurant. Then as mealtime approaches, fill up on healthful foods first.

Some people may use overweight as a defense. A heavy body may fend off intimacy or other anxiety-provoking encounters. The vast majority of overweight people are not in this category, but, if you are, it will be helpful to recognize it.

Are you eating out of boredom? We need many forms of nourishment: friends, intellectual challenges, physical activities, romance, challenges and successes in our lives, rest, and sleep. When these are absent, food may become a cheap substitute. Is food taking the place of something else?

If you are saying, "I overeat, but I do it because food tastes so good," it may be worth examining what else occupies your time. If your life is filled with boredom, then food may well be the most exciting thing in it. It is important to see what prevents you from engaging more fully in other activities that make life what it is.

I would like to refer you to two additional resources. First, Overeaters Anonymous has helped many, many people. Their number is listed in your telephone book. If you really are overeating, OA can be a terrific help. Second, there is a book by Victoria Moran, called *The Love-Powered Diet,** which is entirely devoted to helping people who eat in response to emotions. It has more helpful information on dealing with overeating than any other book I have seen.

3. *Carbohydrate Craving:* There is a group of people who have a particular craving for carbohydrates. It is not because of their taste; the foods can be either sweet or starchy. It is apparently due to an effect carbohydrates have on brain chemistry. Carbohydrates boost a brain chemical called serotonin, which is important in brain functions, including sleep and mood regulation. Most antidepressants increase serotonin levels in the brain, among other actions. One theory is that carbohydrate cravers have naturally low levels of serotonin and, so, tend to be depressed. They eat large quantities of carbohydrates because they have noticed that it helps them to feel better.

That is the theory. Here is the chemistry behind it: Carbohydrates break down in the body to sugars, which, in turn, stimulate insulin secretion. Insulin is a hormone produced in the pancreas. It helps get sugar out of the blood stream and into the cells of the body. Now that is not all insulin does. It also helps amino acids, which are the building blocks of protein, to get out of the blood stream and into the cells. So, after a carbohydrate-rich meal, insulin drives the sugar and the amino acids out of the blood and into the cells.

Now here is the interesting part: As the insulin drives the amino acids out of the blood, it leaves behind one particular amino acid called tryptophan. Tryptophan stays behind because it is stuck to a large carrier molecule. Without all the other amino acids around, tryptophan has less competition for getting into the brain. So the tryptophan passes into the brain, where it is converted to serotonin, which can alter moods, and cause sleepiness.

---

*New World Library/Publishers' Group West, 1992

Carbohydrates Can Aid Sleep
By Increasing Tryptophan In The Brain

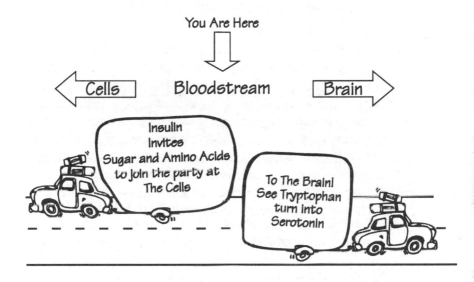

The bottom line is that carbohydrate-rich meals increase serotonin in the brain. Carbohydrate cravers tend to become depressed in the winter months when the days are short. Food may help normalize their brain chemistry.

There is nothing wrong with a high-carbohydrate menu. As we have seen, carbohydrates are very important. The key is to select foods rich in complex carbohydrates, such as rice and other grains, beans, and vegetables, rather than sugar candies or sugar-fat mixtures which really will add to one's waistline.

The Role of Physical Activity

Our lives have become all too sedentary. We have eliminated most of the physical activities that got our blood moving when we were younger and that kept our ancestors fit. It is terrific to bring physical activity back into our lives, for four reasons:

1st   **Movement burns calories**
Every movement you make, whether it is blinking your eyes or lifting a grand piano, burns some calories. The more we move, the more calories we burn.

2nd   **Regular physical activity boosts your metabolism.**
Calories are burned more quickly, not only while you are exercising but also afterward for a period of time.

3rd   **Physical activity helps preserve your muscle mass**
Muscle tissue has a rapid metabolism and is much better than fat tissue at burning off the calories we ingest. If your muscles waste away from inactivity, your body burns fewer calories per hour.

4th   **Physical activity helps control the appetite**
Twenty minutes of exercise before dinner reduces the appetite slightly. This seems to be particularly true for activities that warm the body, such as tennis, running, or dancing (Some people experience an *increase* in appetite after cooling exercises, such as swimming.) Unfortunately, it is likely that overweight people experience less (or even none) of the exercise-induced change in appetite than do normal-weight individuals, so this may be a mechanism that helps people stay thin rather than helping people to get thin.[4]

There are numerous other benefits of physical activity, from reduced risk of heart disease and cancer to more energy and a more relaxed outlook on life. You may find that you will sleep more soundly when your body is tired from exercise. In turn, better sleep makes you feel like taking care of yourself. Chronically tired people prop themselves up with all sorts of indulgences, including unhealthful foods, that do not seem so important when they are well rested.

How Much Activity?

Let's start with a half-hour walk every day, or, if you prefer, an hour three times per week. Pick a place to walk that is enjoyable for you. Enjoy the sights, sounds, and smells.

Feel free to substitute any equivalent activity in place of walking. Here are some examples of physical activities and the number of calories they burn:

Activity	Calories
A brisk half-hour walk:	120
A leisurely half-hour bicycle ride:	140
A half-hour ping-pong game:	210
A half-hour swim:	240
A half-hour jog:	284
An hour of gardening:	300
An hour of golf:	356
An hour of tennis:	456

The key is to have fun. Choose something you'll enjoy.

If you like dancing, gardening, bike-riding, a run with your dog, or a vigorous walk in the woods, then off you go! Bring a friend along if you can. Making activity a social event decreases the possibility of drifting back into sedentary living. At work, use the stairs instead of the elevator.

If you have access to a health club, you will find all sorts of sports and physical activities that turn exercise into pleasure. The old gym has really been transformed into an environment that makes physical activity fun and tailors it to the individual.

Start slowly, particularly if you have been sedentary for some time. If you are over 40 or have any history of illness or joint problems, talk over your plans with your doctor. And remember, stick with activities that you really enjoy.

If you have been on a low-calorie diet, you should switch to a low-fat, high-carbohydrate menu without calorie restriction before you begin any program of regular vigorous exercise. The reason is that the low-calorie diet probably slowed down your metabolism. Even though exercise will boost the metabolic rate of most people, it can actually have the opposite effect on people who have been starving themselves. So stop the calorie restriction first, then, after a couple of weeks, add physical activity.

What About Genetics?

There is one factor we cannot control, and that is our genetic inheritance. Like it or not, if your parents were both thin, you and your siblings will tend to be thin. If your parents were heavy, you will have a similar tendency.

We also tend to inherit our parents' shape. If your parents were apple-shaped, carrying their weight in their chests and abdomens, you are likely to be apple-shaped as well. If they were "pears," carrying their weight in their hips and thighs, you are likely to be pear-shaped as well. There are all sorts of shape variations. Size is more easily changed than shape. If you carry your weight in your hips, as you lose weight you might become a skinny "pear," but you will still be a "pear."

Fat on the abdomen is easier to lose than hip fat. Although hip fat is more difficult to remove, it is also less likely to contribute to health problems. To determine whether you are at greater risk of health problems from being overweight, take a tape measure and measure around your waist and around your hips. For men, increased risk of health problems begins when your waist is bigger than your hips. For women, they begin when your waist is more than 80 percent of your hip measurement.

If you have passed that point, your weight problem is not a cosmetic issue anymore. It is a very real contributor to heart problems, cancer, diabetes, and a broad range of other problems that you do not want to have.

Some people believe that, because there is a strong genetic component to our size and shape, there is nothing they can do to lose weight. This is not true. Although the genetic factors that are passed from parents to children exert important effects, we do not just give our children DNA. We also give them recipes. We give them attitudes about food and preferences for various kinds of food. We also tend to pass along an interest or disinterest in physical activity, and attitudes about health and about how our bodies should look. These can all be modified, if we decide to do so. Whatever hand we have been dealt by our inheritance, there are still steps we can take to change our weight.

The key about genetics is to remember that it is only one of several factors that affect your weight. It shows your tendency. But within that tendency, there is a great deal that you can do to help reach the body size you want.

A Word About B₁₂

Vitamin B₁₂ is needed in minute amounts for healthy blood and healthy nerves. It is not made by plants or animals; it is made by microorganisms, such as bacteria and algae. In traditional societies, B₁₂ is produced by bacteria found in the soil and on vegetables. It also can occur naturally in the process of preparation of foods, such as Asian miso or tempeh, soyfoods which are loaded with the vitamin. In the West, modern hygiene and pasteurization have eliminated these traditional sources. Meat-eaters get the vitamin B₁₂ that bacteria produce in the digestive tracts of animals and passes into the animals' tissues, but people who adhere to a vegetarian diet (as I recommend) should pick up a supplement.

All common multivitamins (One-A-Day, Flintstones, StressTabs, etc.) contain B₁₂. The RDA for B₁₂ is only two micrograms per day. Health food stores carry vegetarian vitamin brands which are free of dairy and meat extracts. Your body has a very good supply

of this vitamin already, but if you have been on a strict vegetarian diet for three years, you should begin taking at least 3 micrograms per day of any common supplement of vitamin B₁₂.

Summary of Basic Concepts

Let's summarize the major points:

Diet: The overall dietary changes are simple.

✦ Eat foods from plant sources: grains, beans, vegetables, and fruits.

✦ Avoid animal products

✦ Keep vegetable oil to a minimum as well.

What these simple steps do is to cut way down on fat, reduce protein content moderately, and give us the metabolic boost of carbohydrates, plus lots of fiber.

✦ Avoid calorie restrictions.

Unless you are really stuffing yourself, you can enjoy unlimited quantities of foods. If you really are overeating, you will need to address the psychological factors that prevent you from treating your body better.

✦ Refined sugars and alcohol should be avoided as well.

It is not necessary to resolve to change your eating habits for the rest of your life. All you can change is what you are doing today. And tomorrow, you can make the same decision again, if you like. But you do not need to plan what you will eat 20 years from now. I point this out because sometimes the idea of life-long change can be frightening. Don't worry about it. *All you need to work on is what you are doing today. And if you like it, you can stick with it.*

To get the results you want, do not water down these guidelines. Adding occasional servings of chicken or french fries will erode your progress. Give yourself the best.

Physical Activity:

✦ Walk for a half-hour per day or an hour three times a week.

Or substitute any equivalent activity. Have fun. The cumulative effect can be enormous.

Part II

Let's Get Started

Let's Get Started

A Step-by-Setp Program

In Part I, we learned the basic concepts. Now it's time to put them into action by tasting new foods, trying new food stores, activating our muscles, and making a solid change in our lives.

Adapting to a new, improved menu is surprisingly easy. It does take a little time, about three to six weeks for a new habit to become routine, but soon you will wonder why you did not try this before.

First, give yourself a pat on the back. You wanted a change for the better, and here you are, well on your way there. You've already covered a lot of ground in learning about slimming down. Now we will put knowledge into practice. Here is how we will proceed:

1st We will throw out all the high-fat foods that have caused so many problems for us.

2nd We will bring in new and interesting foods that are powerful for permanent weight control.

3rd We will set up a simple, effective program of physical activity that will help burn off the pounds.

Planning for Success

One reason this program works is that it provides a very powerful food program, linked with physical activity. But it does more: it takes into account what human beings need in order to make a major change in eating habits.

Let's face it: it's not always easy to change habits. *But certain things make it much easier and much more likely to stick.*

I recently reviewed several major research projects in which people were asked to change their diets. In some of these projects, the participants changed their diets very dramatically, and in others they hardly changed at all. It became very clear that the programs which yielded the most changes were those which had certain things going for them. These factors have been incorporated in this program:

1. *Asking for the degree of change you want.* Doctors or researchers who sell their patients short with weak recommendations get nothing more than they ask for.
2. *Don't just read about foods; taste them as well.* That will be a major focus of this chapter.
3. *Go for maximal reward.* Nothing is more encouraging than success. So this program not only uses foods, it also brings in enjoyable physical activity designed for what people want most: permanent weight control.
4. *Simplicity in foods.* This program is designed to be easy to remember, with no need for charts, measuring, or limiting serving sizes. The two rules of thumb are:

✦Use no animal products.
✦Keep vegetable oils to an absolute minimum.

These simple guidelines are extremely powerful for long-term weight control.

5. *Foods must be enjoyable.* That means quality and quantity. So this program will use tasty foods and no calorie restriction.

6. *Change completely.* Do not tease yourself with foods. Anyone who has tried to change a habit knows about this one. Let's take smoking as an example. If people try only to cut down on smoking, they get essentially nowhere, because the taste for tobacco is always fresh in their minds. It is very easy to increase the frequency of a habit that has not yet been broken. But if they quit completely, they can get some distance between themselves and tobacco and can start a new habit—the habit of being a non-smoker. The same is true of foods. If you have fried chicken or potato chips once a week, then you are constantly teasing yourself with the taste of these very fattening products. If, however, you get away from these foods completely, you allow a new habit to start; you are getting the force of habit working with you, starting a new habit.

7. *Think short-term.* There is no need to make any resolution about what you will do in the distant future. All you can control is what you are doing now. So plan to follow this program for three weeks. At the end of that time, see how you feel. Notice its effect on your waistline. And if you like what you see, you can try it again for another 21 days. If you continue, you will get its full benefit. If you stop, you will lose all your gains. But think short-term; do not burden yourself with feeling the need to make resolutions for the distant future.

8. *Family and friends.* Our families eat with us. They eat the food we prepare or, perhaps, prepare the food we eat. Having them on our side is a terrific boost. When researchers have worked with patients to modify their diets, they have found that including the family makes a tremendous amount of difference. So ask them to join you in this program. Now, they may not feel a need for

any permanent change in their eating habits. And you do not need to ask them to change permanently. All you need to ask them is to join you while you are working on this program. In many cases, they will want to read it with you. That is the ideal. They will benefit from this program, too. This new way of eating not only slims waistlines; it can also lower cholesterol levels, help control blood pressure, help prevent cancer, and prevent many conditions from constipation to varicose veins. At the very least, however, your family and friends must not tempt you with unhealthful foods while you are working through these lessons, and you must not prepare any unhealthful foods for them.

Frequently families get stuck in old habits. They may even want to talk you out of changing and may forecast failure. In that case, you need to have a short sit-down talk. Tell them that if they care about you, they will understand that this is very important to you. They will help and not hinder you. If you have done this with sufficient sincerity, they will be overcome with guilt and will plead for forgiveness. (You might suggest that they can make it up to you by doing your shopping for you.)

Get them to think of it as a three week adventure in eating, including foods from a host of exotic foreign locales. Involve your kids in the kitchen, learning about new foods by helping you prepare them. My previous book, *The Power of Your Plate*, was written for skeptical family members, and you may wish to give a copy to them. For those who do not enjoy reading, a new cassette tape, *Live Longer, Live Better* is also available.

Follow this program to the letter. **Do not "cheat."** You are embarking on a powerful and rewarding program. Give it every chance for maximal success. You deserve no less, and I believe you will be really pleased with the results.

Getting Offending Foods
Out of the House

The first step is to throw out the foods that have been problems in the past and which will get in your way in the future. You can throw them away or give them away, but the key is to get them completely out of the house.

Before you begin, have a meal. It is very difficult for a hungry person to throw any food product away, no matter how unhealthful it may be. Then go on a search and destroy mission for the high-fat, no-fiber foods in your house. Get rid of all of the following:

Any meat, poultry, or fish products
All dairy products, including butter, milk or cream,
                yogurt and cheese.
Margarine
Vegetable oil. (Yes even olive oil.)
All salad dressings other than non-fat dressings
Cookies, cakes, pies and ice cream, other than non-fat
Potato chips
Nuts and nut butters
Sugary candies

You may notice a certain sense of relief as you rid yourself of these unhealthful products. Now we will stock our shelves with foods that will help us have the body we want.

"All offending food this way, please"

Getting to Know New Foods

We are going to go shopping for new kinds of foods and will learn how to prepare them. Don't worry, they are all easy to fix. Our goal for right now is not to be gourmet cooks, but to learn new kinds of foods and to adapt our tastes to a lower-fat menu. If you like, gourmet recipes can come later.

The foods listed on the following pages create a simple beginning menu, but they are important for you to get to know. They are powerful for slimming down. Some are already quite familiar; others may be new. Some will seem very humble, but do not be deceived. They taste terrific and also have an excellent combination of nutritional factors that make them among the most powerful foods for keeping pounds off permanently.

Eat before shopping!

The emphasis in this list is on convenience and simplicity, with minimal preparation time. For example, you will see canned beans, rather than dried beans. Later, you may wish to cook from scratch, instead of using canned varieties. Frozen vegetables are also included for convenience. Their nutritional value is generally good, and better than canned vegetables.

We will start with a one-week menu. The idea is to stock your kitchen with enough healthful foods to give you a good start on adapting to new food tastes. It will also eliminate the need for frequent shopping trips, which are times of vulnerability to unhealthful impulse purchases.

Most of these items are available from any grocery store, but a few are found only at health food stores, as I will indicate. Notice that you do not have to mix any diet powders, and you certainly do not have to go hungry.

Do not go shopping on an empty stomach. If you do, you risk ending up buying anchovy-packed olives and coconut cream pie and avocado swirl-cake and all the other impulse purchases that seduce hungry stomachs.

People with food allergies should obviously skip any food to which they are allergic. If you are on a sodium-restricted diet, look for low-sodium varieties of canned foods, or compensate with less sodium in other foods. Health food stores often stock low-sodium products.

People on prescribed diets should follow this program in consultation with their health care professional. For example, because these foods improve insulin's efficacy, diabetics may need to reduce their insulin use. Similarly, people with high blood pressure may find they need less of their medication as well. Persons with high triglyccrides may need to limit fruit.

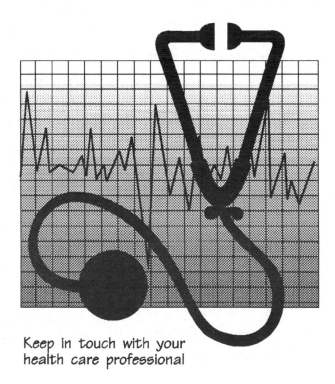

Keep in touch with your
health care professional

First, let's take a look at the foods we will be starting with. Then I will give you a shopping list you can use to guide your trip to the store.

Breakfast

1. **Fresh fruit:** Melon, grapefruit, oranges, bananas, pineapple, or any other fruit you like. It can be your entire breakfast, or just the beginning.
2. **Hot cereal:** Choose from old-fashioned rolled oats, grits, or other hot cereal. Cooked versions are best, but instant is acceptable. If you like, top with cinnamon, or try strawberries, raisins, or other fresh fruit. Do not use milk.
3. **Whole-grain toast.** Have plain, or top with jelly or cinnamon. Do not use butter, margarine, or cream cheese.
4. **Cold cereal with soymilk.** Choose whole-grain cereals. Soymilk is not only free of animal fats; it is also free of the cholesterol and lactose that are found in dairy products. Use only low-fat soymilk, such as Edensoy or Westbrae Lite vanilla flavor (soy milk is carried at any health food store, or in regular groceries near the condensed milks).
5. **Black beans on toast.** This Latin American breakfast sounds unusual, but can be popular on both sides of the border. Simply empty a can of black beans into a saucepan and heat. Spoon the beans onto toast and top with a touch of mild salsa or Dijon mustard. One can of black beans holds two generous servings.
6. **Chick peas (garbanzo beans).** Open a can of chick peas and rinse. Eat plain or with non-fat salad dressing. One can holds two generous servings.

(If you are like me, you will be surprised to see these last two. But try them! You're in for a treat.)

Lunch

At lunch time, convenience is often a key. Low-fat lunches not only help you slim down, they also prevent the after-lunch fatigue that follows high-fat meals.

1. ***Instant soups.*** Health food stores stock a wonderful variety of split pea soup, couscous, noodle soups, and others. These are easy to keep in your desk at work, since you just add hot water. (If you prefer, bring a thermos of vegetable or split pea soup from home.)
2. ***Bread, bread sticks, pretzels, Melba toast.***
3. ***"Finger vegetables"***: cherry tomatoes, baby carrots, broccoli & cauliflower tops with non-fat dressing.
4. ***Fresh fruit:*** Enjoy bananas, apples, pears, oranges, etc., as well as fruit like kiwi and fresh pineapple for a change of pace. Avoid avocados.
5. ***Sandwich:*** Have a CLT: Cucumber, lettuce, and tomato, on whole-grain bread. Add onion and mustard, if you like. Some people like to add sprouts. Unfortunately, most traditional sandwich fillings are loaded with fat. Avoid meats of any kind, cheese, mayonnaise, and peanut butter.
6. ***Chick peas.*** It's easy to keep a can of chick peas in a desk drawer at work. Simply rinse and serve plain, or with non-fat salad dressing.
7. ***Leftovers from dinner or breakfast*** are always welcome. Microwave if you like.
8. ***If you eat lunch in a cafeteria,*** enjoy the cooked vegetables, potatoes, or the salad bar, using a twist of lemon juice instead of dressing. Avoid all meats, eggs, dairy products, and keep vegetable oils to an absolute minimum.

Dinners

In planning meals, I suggest starting with vegetables, usually including two different ones at each meal. Then, add a grain or other starch, such as rice, potatoes, or pasta. Include a bean dish and finish with a serving of fruit. Be generous with grains and other starches, and have smaller portions of bean dishes.

1. ***Vegetables.*** Try broccoli, spinach, carrots, cauliflower, green beans, peas, lima beans, Brussels sprouts, kale, asparagus, succotash, or any other. Any fresh vegetable is fine: spinach leaves, carrots, celery, Boston lettuce or other greens, plus any other salad vegetables that strike your fancy: peppers, tomatoes, cauliflower, etc. If you like, top vegetables with a sprinkle of lemon or lime juice, minced garlic, onion, or parsley. Avoid butter or margarine, sour cream, and other fatty toppings. Do not use oil as a topping or for sautéing or frying. Frozen vegetables are convenient and similar in nutritional value to fresh vegetables. Choose plain varieties, not those in cream sauce.

2. ***Grains and other starches:***
   a. Rice is one of the best foods for slimming down. It is very low in calories and very nutritious. At the grocery store, notice the variety of boxed rice dishes, such as curried rice, long grain and wild rice, brown rice, pecan rice, basmati rice, risotto with tomato, or rice pilaf. Nearby, you will see the fabulous mixes for couscous, tabouli, and vegetarian burgers. Avoid any mixes with meat products or a high fat content. At the health food store, you will find organic short-grain rice, which is an excellent choice (see recipe on page 156). Or try any other varieties of rice that catch your fancy.
   b. Spaghetti with tomato sauce. Whole-grain spaghetti is best. If you are stuck with regular spaghetti,

consider it acceptable for now, even though much of its fiber has been removed. Of commercial tomato sauces, choose those lowest in fat.

c. Bread. Whole-grain varieties are always best.

d. Corn. Corn is a grain, not a vegetable. Enjoy the natural taste of corn without butter, margarine, or oil.

e. Potatoes. Baked, mashed (instant is fine), steamed or boiled. No hash browns, potato chips, or french fries. If you like, a dab of Dijon mustard or ketchup is okay. If you like gravy on potatoes, pick up a can of Franco American Mushroom-Flavor Gravy. Do not add milk to mashed potatoes, and use no butter, sour cream, margarine, cheese, or other fatty toppings.

3. *Legumes (beans, peas, and lentils):*

a. Black beans. Do not skip this one. Black beans are a delightful discovery. They are extremely low in fat, packed with fiber, and delicious. Top with mild salsa or mustard. If you are new to black beans, I strongly suggest buying them canned (note that different brands vary widely in their sodium content), rather than cooking up dried beans, which requires considerably more time. In case you were worrying, for most people, black beans do not seem to cause much gassiness.

b. Vegetarian baked beans. Several canned varieties are available at grocery stores, and are very convenient.

c. Lentil soup. Progresso and other companies make delicious, low-fat lentil soups. For those on sodium-restrictions, health-food stores carry low-sodium varieties.

4. *Fruits.* Pears, cherries, strawberries, peaches, apples, bananas, pineapples and just about any other fruit make great desserts or garnishes for other foods.

Sample Menus

The following menus on page 73 are suggestions for simple starting meals. You can use these, modify them any way you wish (so long as no animal products or vegetable fats are added), or make your own menus from the previous suggestions. You will notice that they are very basic and require almost no preparation time. These will get you started. Note that there is no limit on quantity and you do not need to count calories.

Food Preparation

These basic meals are easy to prepare. Canned beans are simpy heated. Rice, hot cereals, and frozen vegetables are cooked according to package directions. It is easy to cook brown rice from scratch, using the recipe on page 156. Chick peas are simply rinsed and eaten without heating.

You may feel that these foods are too easy; they are very basic. In the next section, we will expand our culinary repertoire to whatever limits you might like. For now, stick with very simple foods as your body learns to enjoy the taste and the benefits of very-low-fat, high-carbohydrate, high-fiber foods.

Sample Menus

Sunday	Monday	Tuesday	Wednesday	Thursday	Friday	Saturday
Breakfast						
melon	grapefruit	orange	melon	orange	melon	grapefruit
oatmeal	oatmeal	cereal & soymilk	cereal & soymilk	black beans on toast	black beans on toast	chick peas
toast	toast					oatmeal
Lunch						
lentil soup	instant soup	CLT (page 58)	chick peas & bread	instant soup	instant soup	instant soup
melba toast	melba toast	carrot sticks	carrot sticks	melba toast	melba toast	melba toast
banana	apple	pear	banana	apple	apple	apple
Dinner						
spaghetti	black beans	chick peas	baked beans	curried rice	lentil soup	black beans
tomato sauce	mild salsa	long & wild rice	potatoes	green beans	baked potatoes	mild salsa
carrots	potato	green beans	corn	spinach	cauliflower	brown rice
peas	broccoli	asparagus	broccoli	chick peas	carrots	broccoli
	spinach with lemon					spinach with lemon

Shopping List

This list supplies two weeks' worth of groceries for one person. It can be multiplied for as many others as necessary.

Canned beans:
>   black beans: 3 cans (low-sodium brands are at health
>   food store)
>   chick peas: 4 cans
>   lentil soup: 2 cans
>   vegetarian baked beans: 2 cans

Cereals and Bread:
>   oatmeal, grits, or other hot cereal: 1 pkg. (regular is
>   preferred, instant is acceptable)
>   cold cereal: one box
>   whole-grain bread: 2 loaves
>   melba toast or bread sticks: 1 pkg.
>   spaghetti: 8 oz.

Rice:
>   long & wild rice: 1 pkg.
>   curried rice: 1 pkg.

Fresh fruits and vegetables:
>   fruit for breakfast (melons, grapefruit, oranges, etc.):
>   5 pieces
>   fruit for lunch (bananas, apples, pears, etc.): 10 pieces
>   fresh carrots (for carrot sticks): 1 small pkg.
>   cucumber: 1
>   lettuce: 1
>   tomatoes: 2
>   potatoes: 3, for baking (or instant potatoes for mashed)
>   lemons: 2, or bottled lemon juice
>   onion: 1
>   or garlic: 1 (optional, for flavoring vegetables)

Frozen vegetables:
 14 packs of frozen vegetables, such as: carrots, cauliflower,
     green beans, corn, peas, broccoli, asparagus, spinach,
     or any others. They are very convenient with nearly
     the same nutritional value as fresh vegetables, but
     you may use fresh vegetables, if you like.

Condiments:
 mild salsa: 1 jar
 Dijon mustard: 1 jar
 jelly (optional, for toast): 1 jar
 cinnamon (optional, for toast or oatmeal)
 raisins (optional, for oatmeal): 1 pkg
 spaghetti sauce: 1 jar (choose brands lowest in fat content)
 Franco American mushroom-flavor gravy: 1 can (optional,
     for potatoes)

Specialty products
 (These are found at any health food store, but may also be
     in the regular grocery)
 soymilk: 1 carton (e.g. Edensoy or Westbrae Lite vanilla, or
     other low-fat brand)
 instant soups: 4 servings. Try split pea, couscous, noodle
     soups, etc.
 low-sodium soy sauce: 1 bottle

While you're at the store, look at the other sauces or condiments: elegant chutneys, mustards, etc. Also see the oil-free salad dressings (Pritikin or other brand) from the dietetic section.

I also suggest picking up a multiple vitamin. Any common brand will do. It does not have to have any special potency, but select a brand without added iron (unless you have a diagnosed iron deficiency.) The goal is simply to cover any vitamin deficiencies you may have gotten on past diets, and to insure a good source of vitamin B_{12}, which is sometimes of concern. If you have been on a pure vegetarian diet for three years or more, you should supplement with vitamin B_{12}. As noted on page 56, this is very easy to do.

Even if you found all you need at the regular grocery store, do stop by the health food store in your area. You will be delighted by the variety of wonderful products that are now available only at these specialty stores. Skip the stores that sell only vitamin supplements.

Check for Overeating

As we said earlier, most overweight people do not overeat. Most actually eat less than thin people. But some people do consume very large amounts of food, not because their bodies need them, but for psychological reasons. From the discussion in Part I, you already know if this includes you.

If it does, now is the time to address this challenge squarely. First, look in the phone book for the nearest Overeaters Anonymous. Many, many people have been helped by OA. Second, pick up a copy of *The Love-Powered Diet,* by Victoria Moran, who has an understanding of compulsive over-eating as one who has been there. It is possible to learn to deal with the emotional rollercoasters of life without plunging into self-destructive habits, and even to smooth out the hills and valleys a bit.

Plan Physical Activity

Now for the easy part. Plan to walk for a half-hour per day or an hour three times per week. That's all you have to do. If you like, you can substitute any equivalent activity.

Do not overdo it. Lots of people start an exercise program much too aggressively and soon become weary of it or feel defeated by it. So we are not even going to use the word "exercise." The point is to enjoy the use of your body so you will want to keep it up. So we are just going to walk or, if you prefer, bike, play tennis, go dancing, or anything equivalent to a good vigorous walk.

First, take a moment, and think about your schedule. When is a time that you can reliably break free from your schedule? Evening? Early morning? Late afternoon? Which is better for you—daily or three times per week? Is there another activity you would like to substitute some or all of the time?

Second, is there someone you can take with you? If not, do not despair. Plenty of spouses and friends have different health practices. But activities that are social are easier to stick with.

Finally, see your doctor before starting an exercise program if you are over forty or have any health problem.

Part III

Moving Into High Gear

Moving Into High Gear

A Step-by-Step Program

Now you have dramatically cut the fat content of your diet, and boosted the carbohydrate and fiber content. This encourages a steady and permanent weight loss, which is improved with exercise. In effect, if your fat stores were a huge bag of water, you just poked a small hole in it. Slowly and surely it will drain out.

In this chapter we will move beyond the simple meals we discussed in Part II, and have a look at how to bring an essentially limitless variety of foods and new food ideas into your life. We will also deal with some of the pitfalls that can sometimes get in our way.

New Recipes, New Foods

First, let's open the doors to new kinds of foods. The variety of healthful foods is enormous, thanks to the many countries that have had culinary traditions very different from our own and to the ever-growing interest in nutrition.

Eating Out

When choosing restaurants, the best ones for low-fat, vegetarian foods are Chinese, Japanese, and other Asian cuisines, Middle-eastern, Indian, Mexican, and Italian. Traveling is a time of challenges to those trying to eat in a healthful way, but many fast-food restaurants have responded to the demand with baked potatoes and salad bars. Taco restaurants feature bean burritos, and the turnpikes of the East Coast even feature spaghetti restaurants in their travel plazas. In your car, bring some fresh fruit or sandwiches along. When you book a flight request a vegetarian meal or fruit plate; all airlines now have them.

Collecting New Recipes

The next time you get a chance, browse through the cookbook section of your local bookstore. There is an astounding wealth of new cookbooks, particularly those offering vegetarian cuisine. They are a goldmine of food ideas. Look at the wonderful pastas, Middle-eastern foods, Asian foods, and on and on. Some use dairy products or more than minimal amounts of oil, but these recipes can often be modified, as noted on page 84. If you have not already seen my earlier book, *The Power of Your Plate*, I would strongly recommend it as a source of in-depth information on a broad range of nutrition issues, as well as many of my own favorite recipes.

New Food Products

Exploring new food products can be delightful as well. Take a look at the health food store. There is a wonderful range of new products, from soups of every variety, dips, and sandwich fillings to exotic entrees that are a snap to prepare. New brands of tortilla chips are baked rather than fried and, so, are oil-free. Many varieties of rice and other grains produced without chemical treatments are there. Delightful beverages are now available ranging from flavored waters to juices and teas.

There is also a huge range of non-meat "transition foods"—foods that take the place of ice cream, mayonnaise, hot dogs, hamburgers, and most other fatty, cholesterol-packed foods. These substitutes are not always good for everyday use, however. While better than the items they imitate, they are often still rather high in fat.

Resource Groups

If there is a vegetarian society in your area, get in touch with them. They have been exploring healthful eating for years, and can be a great source of information.

Tune Up Your Menu

In the last chapter, we brought high-fiber, high-carbohydrate foods to the center of the plate. Now, let's fine-tune things a bit:

Whole grains:

Let whole grains (as opposed to processed grains) play a greater role in your diet. "Processed" grains are ground (e.g. flour) or have some of the fiber removed (e.g. white rice). Evidence indicates that whole grains release a bit fewer of their calories. So rice, rolled oats, or corn may release even fewer calories than flour made from whole grains. Let rice replace bread.

Raw foods:

Be increasingly generous with raw vegetables and fruits. Many people report remarkable weight reductions when they include large amounts of raw fruits and vegetables in their diets. This is partly because these foods are extremely low in fat and high in fiber and carbohydrate, but there may be other contributors that science has not yet unraveled. People with even stubborn weight problems have benefited greatly by eating more raw vegetables and fruits.

When you select raw vegetables, skip the iceberg lettuce; it's mostly water. For a salad, try fresh spinach and the other delightful greens in the produce department. Add peppers, broccoli, celery, carrots, cauliflower, cooked chickpeas, or whatever else you might like. Happily, it is now easier to find vegetables produced without pesticides.

Again, skip dressings that include oil. Enjoy the taste of vegetables without added flavorings.

Modifying recipes:

Recipes that are high in fat can often be easily modified to lower fat content. You will note that often the amounts of oil added to recipes are quite arbitrary. Once you have "re-set" your taste for fat, you will automatically want to leave the grease out of the foods you prepare.

Health food stores sell egg replacer that does exactly that, drastically cutting down the fat content of baked goods. An egg-sized piece of tofu will also accomplish much the same thing in a baking recipe. TVP (texturized vegetable protein), a de-fatted soy product sold at health food stores, replaces ground beef so well that many pizza companies and other ground beef users have already made the switch.

For fat-free frying:

If you are sautéing in oil, here's a helpful tip: Let's say your recipe for spaghetti sauce calls for sautéing onions and garlic in olive oil. How many calories are there in three tablespoons of olive oil? Would you believe 360? Instead, try this: put a half-cup of water in a sauce pan and sauté your onions and garlic in simmering water. You get no extra calories and a pleasant, lighter taste.

The new non-stick pans work remarkably well with this method.

Activity and Rest

Increase physical activity naturally. If you are comfortable with your current level of physical activity, let the time you give it increase naturally. Do not force it, or it will become a chore. But let yourself enjoy an extra night out dancing or bowling, a day on the golf course, or walking in the park. The keys, again, are *fun* and *frequency*.

Get plenty of sleep. People need rest. Chronically tired people have no energy to exercise. Often they feel so out of sorts that they are tempted to prop up their flagging spirits with food or alcohol. There is no substitute for adequate sleep.

Troubleshooting

If you have had insufficient results so far, be patient; slow weight loss is more likely to be permanent than rapid weight loss.

But if you did not lose weight at all, then let's review the basics:

✦ Were you using any oily foods, such as salad dressings, peanut butter, or margarine?

✦ Are you buying fatty products, such as tofu hotdogs?

✦ Were there any animal products in your foods?

✦ How about alcohol?

✦ Did you miss out on regular physical activity?

If you had problems in any of these areas, now is the time to address the problem squarely. There are always solutions to these problems, and tremendous rewards when you do.

Are you having trouble sticking to healthful foods with friends? It may be that you are looking to others for approval, and afraid that they will not sympathize with your new and healthful way of eating. If so, I have noticed a remarkable thing in the past few years. Every time the subject of vegetarian foods comes up in conversation, or I ask a waiter for a vegetarian entree, such as a vegetable plate or spaghetti when there was not one on the menu, I always find that they already know that this is a very healthful way to eat. Many are already vegetarians themselves, or at least recognize that they should be. So stop worrying.

When eating out with friends, suggest Italian, Chinese, or Mexican restaurants. At American-style restaurants, do not hesitate to ask for a vegetable plate. The National Restaurant Association asked all its members in 1991 to feature vegetarian entrees, because, at that time, about one in five diners looked for them. If you don't see it on the menu, by all means ask.

When I am invited to a party, I always say something along the lines of "I am a vegetarian, and I don't want to put you to any trouble. How about if I bring along something like a meatless spaghetti sauce or hummus?" Invariably, my offer is declined, because they planned to have a meatless dish or two. Often, they say that their son or husband is a vegetarian, and it is no problem at all.

Some people have digestive troubles. Any major change in diet can be a temporary challenge for the digestive tract. A meat-eater who becomes a vegetarian suddenly has to adapt to a high-fiber diet. If a vegetarian were to become a meat-eater, a similar problem would occur due to the enormous change in the dietary contents. Any change can lead to temporary indigestion or gas. If this happens to you, be aware that the effect is a temporary price you are paying for your past indiscretions.

Some plant foods—certain varieties of beans, in particular— do tend to cause gas. Try to pin down which is the problem food. Pinto beans, for example, may be a problem, while black beans are not. Include more grains in the diet, such as rice, and deemphasize beans. A new product, called Beano, is sold at health food stores and is reported to eliminate the gassy effect of foods.

Good Luck!

This program is so elegantly simple, yet it is the most effective way to control your weight permanently. The great part is that there is no need to count calories, skip meals, or eat small portions. You can enjoy food in reasonable quantities, and enjoy it in a slimmer, healthier body.

I hope you will let me know how this program works for you. Please write to me at the Physicians Committee for Responsible Medicine. PCRM can also keep you posted on the latest in nutrition through our magazine, *Good Medicine.*

Let me wish you the very best of health and success in your new venture.

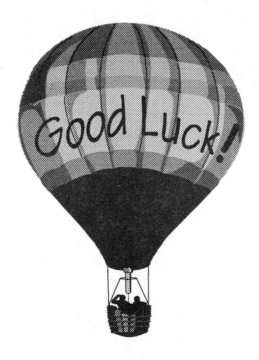

References

[1]Foster GD, et al. Controlled trial of the metabolic effects of a very-low-calorie diet: short-and long-term effects. Am J Clin Nutr 1990;51:167-72.

[2]Chen J, Campbell TC, Junyao L, Peto R. Diet, life-style, and mortality in China. 1990, Oxford University Press, Oxford.

[3]de Castro JM, Orozco S. Moderate alcohol intake and spontaneous eating patterns of humans: evidence of unregulated supplementation. Am J Clin Nutr 1990;52:246-253.

[4]Kissileff HR, Pi-Sunyer FX, Segal K, Meltzer S, Foelsch PA. Acute effects of exercise on food intake in obese and nonobese women. Am J Clin Nutr 1990;52:240-5.

Part IV

Menus and Recipes

Day 1

Breakfast — ¼ cantaloupe
³/₄ cup cooked oatmeal
    with raisins and cinnnamon
1 slice whole grain bread, toasted

Lunch — 1 slice *Vegetable Pizza, page 150*
2 cups *Mixed Green Salad, page 128*
    with *Fat Free Herb Salad Dressing, page 128*
1 medium apple

Dinner — 1 cup *Vegetable Chop Suey, page 149*
    on ³/₄ cup *Brown Rice, page 156*
mashed butternut squash
½ cup fresh strawberries

Day 2

Breakfast — 1 sliced orange
³/₄ cup prepared cereal
    with ¼ cup blueberries
    and ¼ cup light soymilk

Lunch — 1 cup *Split Pea Soup, page 122*
2 *Bread Sticks, page 107*
1 cup *Cabbage-Pineapple Slaw, page 125*
½ cup unsweetened applesauce

Dinner — 2 *Spicy Lentil Patties, page 146*
1 slice whole grain gread
1 cup fresh asparagus
carrot sticks
½ cup *Orange-Banana Compote, page 172*

Day 3

Breakfast — 1 large slice melon
$^3/_4$ cup prepared cereal
    with $^1/_4$ cup light soymilk
1 *Raisin English Muffin*, page 109, toasted

Lunch — 2 cups *Mixed Green Salad*, page 128
    with *Fat Free Herb Salad Dressing*, page 128
1$^1/_2$ cups *Vegetarian Chili*, page 151
2 *Bread Sticks*, page 107
1 medium plum

Dinner — 2 slices *Tofu Meatless Loaf*, page 148
    or *Lentil Bulghur Loaf*, page 145
1 cup mashed potatoes
    with $^1/_2$ cup *Mushroom Gravy*, page 159
1 cup cooked green beans
1 *Baked Apple*, page 166
(Mash the potatoes with cooking liquid to moisten)

Day 4

Breakfast — $^1/_2$ grapefruit
$^3/_4$ cup hot cereal
    with raisins & cinnamon
2 slices *Holiday Fruit Braid*, page 112

Lunch — 1 cup *Cabbage Potato Soup*, page 118
1 cup *Colorful Couscous Salad with Chick Peas*,
    page 126
1 *Herbed Yeast Roll*, page 110
1 slice melon

Dinner — 3 *Oat Mushroom Patties*, page 147
1 cup *Hot Broccoli and Potato Salad*, page 127
1 small tomato, sliced
$^1/_2$ cup *Fruit Salad*, page 170

Day 5

Breakfast — ½ grapefruit
1 cup black beans
1 slice whole grain bread, toasted

Lunch — Hearty Vegetable Soup, page 119
½ cup Lentil Paté, page 99, on melba toast
1 medium peach or apple

Dinner — 1 cup Vegetable Chop Suey, page 149
 on 1 cup Brown Rice, page 156
1 cup Zucchini Salad, page 130
2 Fruit Kabobs, page 169

Day 6

Breakfast — ⅙ honeydew melon
¾ cup prepared cereal
¼ cup light soymilk
1 toasted Raisin English Muffin, page 109

Lunch — 1 cup Black Bean Soup, page 117
2 Sesame Herb Crackers, page 111
2 cups Mixed Green Salad, page 128
 with Fat Free Herb Salad Dressing, page 128
1 medium pear

Dinner — 1 cup Curried Lentils, page 144
 on ¾ cup Brown Rice, page 156
2 Tbsp. Ginger Pear Chutney, page 157
1 cup Cabbage-Pineapple Slaw, page 125
¾ cup broccoli or Brussel sprouts
½ cup Fruit Salad, page 170

Day 7

Breakfast —
1 slice melon in season
2 slices Holiday Fruit Braid, page 112
$3/4$ cup cooked oatmeal
  with cinnamon & raisins

Lunch —
1 cup Lentil Vegetable Soup, page 121
2 Sesame Herb Crackers, page 111
1 cup broccoli
1 small banana

Dinner —
1 cup Hearty Pinto Bean Stew, page 143
  on $3/4$ cup Brown Rice, page 156
1 cup cooked zucchini
2 cups Mixed Green Salad, page 128
  with Fat Free Herb Salad Dressing, page 128
Baked Apple, page 166

Snack Suggestions

Save a fruit from one of the menus to eat mid-afternoon or as an evening snack. Or choose one:

3 cups air popped popcorn
1 cup carrot sticks
1 small cucumber, cut in sticks
1 medium apple
1 medium peach
$1/2$ cup Fruit Salad, page 170
$1/2$ cup Orange-Banana Compote, page 172

APPETIZERS

Lentil Paté

Makes 3 ½ cups

Cut **8 slices rye bread** into small cubes (should be 2 cups, packed).

Pour over bread:
1 cup hot vegetable stock

Let bread soak while cooking lentils. Combine in pan:
2½ cups water
1 cup brown lentils, washed
3 cloves garlic, cut up
1 bay leaf
½ tsp. salt

Bring lentils to a boil, reduce heat, cover and cook 35-40 minutes until tender. Liquid should be absorbed, but lentils should be moist. Remove bay leaf.

While lentils cook, sauté in a hot skillet:
1 onion, chopped fine
1 tsp. dark sesame oil
2 tsp. fresh ginger, minced

When onions are soft, sprinkle with:
1 Tbsp. soy sauce
1 tsp. marjoram
1 tsp. thyme
pinch of cayenne

Mix onions with the lentils and puree in blender or food processor. Mix well with the soaked bread cubes. Heat oven to 350°. Taste paté and add a little salt if desired. Pack into a well-oiled round quart pan. Cover with foil. Place pan in a larger pan of hot water. Bake 45 minutes, remove foil, bake 15 minutes more. Cool 30 minutes, run a knife around sides of pan to loosen and invert loaf on serving plate.

Serve paté with melba toast.

BREAKFAST

Rice Barley Cream Cereal

6 servings

Wash, drain, cover with water and soak overnight:
> **1 cup barley**

Wash well:
> **2 cups brown rice**

Combine grains with:
> **5 cups water**
> **pinch of salt**

Bring to a boil. Turn heat to low and simmer 50 minutes. It should have a creamy consistency.

Sprinkle on as a garnish:
> **2 tsp. sunflower seeds, toasted**

BREADS

Bread Sticks

Makes 24 sticks

Place in a bowl and let stand 5 minutes:
   1 Tbsp. yeast
   1 tsp. barley malt
   ¹/₄ cup warm water

Add:
   3 cups whole wheat flour
   ³/₄ cup warm water
   1 Tbsp. oil
   2 Tbsp. nutritional yeast (opt.)
   ¹/₂ tsp. salt

Mix dough until it forms a ball, then knead 10 minutes until smooth. Oil a bowl, turn dough around to coat, then cover dough and let rise until double. Press dough down, break off 24 pieces. Roll each into a stick about 8" long. If desired, roll sticks in sesame or caraway seeds. Place on oiled baking sheet. Cover with waxed paper and let rise again. Bake at 400° for 5 minutes, turn over with tongs, bake 5 to 7 minutes more.

Variation:

Onion Twists

Chop 1 onion finely, sauté in the oil before mixing with the dough. Twist each stick.

Brown Rice Sesame Bread

Makes 1 loaf (20 slices)

A hearty, dense yeast-free bread. Using grains in bread requires fermenting time which varies with the seasons. Dough will be sticky, knead with wet hands.

Combine in a bowl and mix well:

3 cups whole wheat flour
1 cup cornmeal
¹/₄ tsp. salt
¹/₂ cup unhulled roasted sesame seeds

Add and work in your hands:

1¹/₄ cups cooked short grain brown rice

Spread the mixture out to make a well in the center, add:

1¹/₄ cups warm water

Mix with a wooden spoon, adding a little more water if needed to make a moist bread dough. Knead for about 15 minutes, until dough comes together. It will be sticky. Have ready a well-oiled bowl. Place dough in bowl and turn over twice to coat with oil. Lightly oil a sheet of waxed paper and place oiled side down on top of dough. Cover bowl with camp towel. Keep in a cool place for 13 to 15 hours in the summer, 24-26 hours in winter. Place dough in an oiled loaf pan, making a dash down the center of the loaf with a sharp knife. Place pan in a cold oven. Turn heat to 200° and bake for 25 minutes. Raise heat to 350° and bake 1 hour. Loaf should be well browned and starting to pull away from sides of pan. Cool.

Raisin English Muffins

Makes 12 4" muffins

Place in a large bowl to foam:

¹/₄ cup warm water
2 Tbsp. yeast
1 tsp. maple syrup

Stir in:

4 cups whole wheat flour (or half unbleached flour)
1 cup water
1 Tbsp. safflower oil
¹/₂ tsp. salt
¹/₂ cup raisins
¹/₂ tsp. cinnamon

Knead dough 10 minutes on a floured work surface. Roll out and cut into a dozen 4" rounds. Dust a baking sheet with cornmeal, place muffins on sheet. Let rise for 1 hour in a warm place. Bake 350° for about 25 minutes.

Herbed Yeast Rolls

Makes 24 rolls

Let stand for 5 minutes:

1 Tbsp. yeast
¹/₂ cup warm water
1 Tbsp. barley malt

Stir in one cup warm water:

3 cups whole wheat flour
3 cups unbleached white flour
1 Tbsp. safflower oil
1 tsp. oregano
¹/₂ tsp. salt
¹/₂ tsp. thyme
¹/₂ tsp. dill

Mix until a ball of dough forms. Knead dough on lightly floured surface until elastic. Oil a bowl lightly, turn dough around to coat, cover with a damp towel and let rise in a warm place until double. Knead down and pull apart to form small balls. Grease 2 dozen muffin tins. Place 3 small balls in each section to make cloverleafs. Cover pans. Let rise until almost double, about 1 hour. Bake at 375° for about 20 minutes. Remove from tins and serve while hot.

Sesame Herb Crackers

Makes 3 dozen

Mix together:
- **2 cups whole wheat flour**
- **¹/₄ cup sesame seeds**
- **2 Tbsp. wheat germ**
- **2 Tbsp. bran**
- **¹/₂ tsp. each of oregano, basil, garlic powder, dried parsley**

Stir in:
- **³/₄ cup cold water**
- **1 Tbsp. sesame oil**

Roll dough out onto a lightly oiled cookie sheet or roll thinly between two pieces of waxed paper and transfer to sheet. Cut into squares or diamond shapes before baking. Bake in a preheated oven at 400° for 15-20 minutes. Cool, break apart.

Variation

Substitute ¹/₄ cup onion flakes for the bran and wheat germ.

Holiday Fruit Braid

1 large loaf (20 slices)

*A beautiful and delicious bread that can be made ahead,
as the fruit keeps it from drying out.*

Bring to a boil in a small saucepan:

1 cup dried papaya, snipped small with a scissors
¹/₂ cup dried apricots, snipped small
¹/₂ cup raisins
1 cup water

Cover, remove from heat and let stand 15 minutes.

Combine in a large bowl:

1 Tbsp. yeast
¹/₄ cup warm water
1 Tbsp. safflower oil
2 Tbsp. maple syrup

Mix and add:

2 tsp. finely shredded lemon peel
¹/₄ tsp. nutmeg
¹/₄ tsp. mace

Drain liquid from the dried fruit into a measuring cup and add
enough water to make 1 cup liquid. Add to yeast and
seasonings.

Stir in:

3¹/₂ cups whole wheat pastry flour

Add more flour as needed to make a firm dough, working in
the dried fruit, kneading bread about 10 minutes. Oil a bowl
and turn dough around in it to coat. Cover with a damp towel
and put in a warm place until double in bulk (1 to 1¹/₂ hours).
Press dough down, divide into 4 balls. Lightly oil a baking
sheet. Roll and stretch 3 of the balls into long ropes and braid
these on the sheet. Divide remaining ball into 3 pieces and

make the 3 smaller ropes into a braid, laying this on top of large braid. Let rise 45 minutes to 1 hour. Preheat oven to 350° and bake 35 to 40 minutes. Remove from pan and cool. Decorate if desired: press pieces of dried fruit (such as dried pineapple or papaya) on top in any pattern you like.

SOUPS

Black Bean Soup

Makes 6 servings

Wash, drain, cover with water and soak overnight or for 8 hours:

1¹/₂ cups black beans

Drain beans. Add, and bring to boil:

6 cups water

Cover, simmer for 1 hour. Add:

3 cloves garlic, smashed
2 small onions, cut in wedges
3 small carrots, cut chunky
2 stalks celery, sliced thinly

Cook about 30 minutes until beans are tender. Stir in:

2 Tbsp. apple cider vinegar
2 Tbsp. soy sauce
2 tsp. cumin
2 tsp. oregano

Cook 10 minutes to blend flavors. Serve with a scoop of brown rice, if desired, garnish with copped red onions.

Cabbage Potato Soup

Makes 6 servings

Place in a 3 quart pan and bring to a boil:

4 potatoes, cut in 1" chunks
4 cups water
1 large onion, chopped
1 tsp. salt

Reduce heat to low, simmer 15 minutes. Heat skillet and add:

$^1/_2$ tsp. safflower oil
$^1/_2$ head cabbage, chopped (about 4 cups)

Sauté until tender, add to soup and simmer 5 minutes. With a slotted spoon, remove about a cup of the cooked potatoes to a soup bowl and mash with a fork. Stir mashed potato into soup to thicken it, stir in:

$^1/_2$ cup soymilk
$^1/_4$ cup parsley

Cook slowly a few minutes to heat milk but do not boil.

Hearty Vegetable Soup

6 servings

Rinse and drain:

1 cup brown rice

Add to a large kettle with:

6 cups water
1 rutabaga, diced
1 sweet potato, chopped
1 white turnip, diced
1 medium onion, cut in chunks
2 carrots, cut in chunks

Bring to a boil, lower heat, cover and cook on medium low heat for 45 minutes. Add 1 to 2 cups water if too thick.

Add:

2 cups chopped kale, well rinsed

Cook 15 minutes. Ladle into bowls.

Leek Soup

6 servings

Chop bottoms ends off:
2 large leeks

Wash ends, boil 10 minutes for stock with:
6 cups water

Remove and discard ends. Clean rest of leeks carefully and slice into 1" pieces.

Return the chopped leeks to kettle and simmer for 15—20 minutes until tender along with:
1 celery stalk with leaves, chopped
2 small carrots, sliced, cut in half
2 scallions, chopped (optional)
1 cup sliced mushrooms

Before heat is turned off, add:
1 Tbsp. soy sauce

Top each bowl with minced parsley.

Lentil Vegetable Soup

Makes 8 servings

Combine in a soup pot:

2 cups brown lentils, washed and drained
8 cups water
1 cup onion, chopped
¹/₂ cup carrot, chopped
¹/₂ cup celery, chopped
2 cloves garlic, minced

Bring to a boil, lower heat, cover and simmer 1 hour. Add:

2 cups tomatoes (16 oz. can), chopped
¹/₄ cup parsley, minced
2 Tbsp. apple cider vinegar
1 tsp. oregano

Cook another 30 minutes.

Split Pea Soup

6 servings

Rinse split peas, then combine with water and vegetables:

2 cups green split peas
1 onion, chopped
2 carrots, chopped into chunks
6 cups water

Cook 45 minutes until peas are tender. Stir in:

1 tsp. ginger powder
1 tsp. thyme
1 Tbsp. soy sauce

Simmer a few minutes.

SALADS

Cabbage-Pineapple Slaw

Makes 1 quart

Mix in a bowl:
4 cups cabbage, shredded
1 large carrot, grated
1 small can (8 oz.) unsweetened pineapple tidbits with juice
2 Tbsp. cider vinegar

Cover and chill.

Colorful Couscous Salad with Chick Peas

8 servings

Bring to a boil:

3 cups water

Stir in, cover and remove from heat:

2 cups couscous

Let sit 5 minutes, fluff with a fork, turn into large mixing bowl to cool.

Add:

2 cups cooked chick peas, chopped
1 carrot, thinly sliced
1 red pepper, chopped
¹/₄ cup currants, soaked in 2 Tbsp. hot water
2 Tbsp. parsley, chopped
2 Tbsp. red onion, chopped

For dressing, stir in a small bowl:

2 Tbsp. lemon juice
¹/₄ cup olive oil
1 Tbsp. apple cider vinegar
2 tsp. brown rice syrup
1 tsp. Dijon mustard
¹/₂ tsp. salt

Stir dressing into salad.

Hot Broccoli and Potato Salad

6 servings

Steam or cook in a small amount of boiling water until just tender:

5 new potatoes, medium size, cut into bite-size chunks

Drain and keep warm.

Wash, peel stems and cut into bite-size pieces:

1 lb. broccoli

Steam stems and flower until crisp tender. Combine in a small pan, bring to a boil, then remove from heat:

2 Tbsp. olive oil
3 Tbsp. apple cider vinegar
1 tsp. soy sauce
3 Tbsp. parsley, minced
2 cloves garlic, minced

Stir into dressing:

3 green onions, sliced with tops
¼ tsp. cayenne

Arrange potatoes and broccoli on a serving platter and pour hot mixture over them. Garnish with cherry tomatoes.

Mixed Green Salad

Toss with ¼ cup *Fat Free Herb Dressing* until every leaf
glistens.

**2 cups torn romaine
2 cups torn iceberg lettuce
1 cup spinach leaves
1 cucumber, sliced
1 rib celery, thinly sliced
6 radishes, sliced
½ red onion, diced**

Optional additions:

Sliced fresh mushrooms, strips of red, green or yellow
    peppers, flowerets of broccoli or cauliflower, thin slices
    of zucchini or yellow squash.

Fat Free Herb Salad Dressing

Makes ½ cup.

Shake up in a small jar.

**¼ cup cider vinegar
¼ cup unsweetened apple juice
½ tsp. each: onion powder, oregano, basil, dill, dry
    mustard
¼ tsp. lemon pepper**

Tabouli (Bulghur Wheat)

6 servings

Adding beans to a grain makes a complete protein meal.

Let soak for 30 minutes or until water is absorbed:
1 cup boiling water
1 cup bulghur.

Stir in:
1 cup cooked chick peas
4 green onions, chopped
1 tomato, chopped
1 red pepper, chopped
2 cloves garlic, minced
1 cucumber, chopped
¼ cup parsley, minced
1 Tbsp. olive oil
juice of 1 lemon
chopped fresh mint or basil

Toss well and chill and serve on lettuce.

Zucchini Salad

6 servings

Have ready in a bowl:

2 medium zucchini, sliced
2 cups cabbage, shredded
$^1/_2$ cup celery, sliced
$^1/_4$ cup red onion, diced

Cook in a small pan for just 1 minute:

$^1/_4$ cup barley malt syrup
$^1/_4$ cup cider vinegar
2 tsp. celery seed
$^1/_4$ tsp. salt

Pour dressing over vegetables, toss and serve.

VEGETABLES

Gingered Chick Peas and Kale

6 servings

Wash, drain and soak overnight in 4 cups water:
1 cup uncooked chick peas

Drain and rinse peas, add 4 cups water and cook 1 to 1½ hours until tender. Drain again, and keep warm.

Heat skillet and sauté:
1 Tbsp. fresh ginger, chopped
1 tsp. safflower oil
1 onion, chopped

Add chick peas and:
¾ lb. kale, cooked
2 Tbsp. soy sauce
1 Tbsp. cider vinegar

Serve over cooked brown rice or noodles.

Mixed Vegetable with Lemon Sauce

6 servings

Heat in a large pan and add:
>**1 cup onion, chopped**
>**3 cloves garlic**
>**1 cup water**
>**2 cups broccoli flowers**
>**¹/₂ cup zucchini, chopped**
>**¹/₂ cup carrot, chopped**

Cover and simmer until crisp tender. Add:
>**¹/₄ cup lemon juice**
>**2 Tbsp. soy sauce**
>**1 tsp. grated lemon rind**

Mix together, then stir into vegetables:
>**3 Tbsp. whole wheat flour**
>**¹/₄ cup cold water**

Cook until sauce thickens. Serve over brown rice or pasta.

Sprouts with Sesame Sauce

6 servings

Rinse and drain:

> **1 lb. fresh bean sprouts. (Mung bean or lentil sprouts are best.)**

Cut into 1" sticks and parboil for 30 seconds, then drain:

> **1 large carrot**

Chop:

> **2 green onions with tops**

Toast in hot dry skillet until they begin to pop:

> **2 Tbsp. sesame seeds**

Place seeds in a bowl with:

> **¹/₄ cup brown rice syrup**
> **1 Tbsp. soy sauce**
> **2 Tbsp. cider vinegar**
> **1 tsp. sesame oil**

Mix sauce, then toss with sprouts, carrots and onions.

Stuffed Baked Tomatoes

6 servings

Wash, scoop out hollow on stem end, remove pulp, leaving shell:

6 medium tomatoes

Simmer:

3 Tbsp. water
¹/₂ cup onion, chopped
¹/₂ cup red pepper, chopped
¹/₂ cup green onions, chopped

Mix together:

tomato pulp, mashed
1 cup cooked brown rice
¹/₂ cup parsley, chopped
1 Tbsp. soy sauce
1 Tbsp. basil
pinch of cayenne

Combine cooked vegetables with rice mixture. Stuff tomatoes and place in lightly oiled baking pan. Bake at 375° for 20-25 minutes.

Sweet Potato Tangerine Casserole

6 servings

Steam until tender, then cut into 1" slices:
6 medium sweet potatoes, scrubbed

Peel and separate into segments:
4 seedless tangerines

Combine in a sauce pan:
$^1/_2$ cup brown rice or maple syrup
$^1/_2$ cup apple juice
$^1/_2$ cup water
1 Tbsp. cornstarch

Cook over low heat until thickened, stirring. In an oiled casserole, arrange layers of potatoes and tangerines.

Sprinkle with:
$^1/_2$ tsp. cinnamon

Pour sauce over, bake at 350° for 30 minutes.

ENTREES

Barley Pilaf

4 servings

Simmer for 1 hour:

3 cups vegetable stock or water
1 cup barley
¹/₄ tsp. salt

Simmer in small skillet:

3 Tbsp. water
1 onion, sliced
1 carrot, chopped
1 stalk celery, chopped
¹/₂ cup green onion, sliced

Stir vegetables into the cooked barley, adding:

1 Tbsp. soy sauce
1 tsp. thyme

Simmer the pilaf for 5 minutes, until liquid is absorbed.

Serve with:

fresh parsley or kale for garnish

Chick Peas and Carrot Sauce

4 servings

Wash, drain, cover with water and soak overnight:
1 cup chick peas

Rinse again and bring to a boil with:
4 cups water

Cover reduce heat and simmer 1 to 1½ hours, until tender.

Heat a 2 quart saucepan and sauté:
1 Tbsp. sesame oil
2 carrots, cut in chunks
1 large onion, cut in wedges
1 Tbsp. fresh ginger, chopped fine

Remove half the chick peas to a bowl and mash. Add to onions with remaining chick peas and the cooking liquid. Cover and simmer until vegetables are tender.

Stir in:
2 Tbsp. cornstarch dissolved in ¼ cup cold water
pinch of salt

Cook, stirring until thickened. Blend in:
1 Tbsp. soy sauce
½ cup chopped parsley

Serve over couscous or rice.

Hearty Pinto Bean Stew

6 servings

Wash, drain, cover with water and soak overnight:
1 cup pinto beans

Drain again, add and bring to a boil with:
5 cups water

Cover, reduce heat, simmer 1 hour until tender.

Sauté together:
2 tsp. sesame oil
2 onions, cut in large wedges
2 tsp. fresh ginger, minced

After 5 minutes, add:
2 carrots, cut in wedges
1 parsnip, cut in chunks

Sauté 5 minutes. Add vegetables to beans and cook until beans are tender. Remove 1 cup cooked beans, mash, stir in a little of the cooking liquid and:
2 Tbsp. soy sauce

Stir well and return to pan. Let simmer 10 minutes, stirring occasionally. Mashed beans should give a gravy consistency. Taste for seasonings.

Serve on brown rice, garnish with minced parsley.

Curried Lentils

4 servings

Double this recipe for a company dish.

Rinse lentils and cook 35-40 minutes until soft:

1 cup lentils
5 cups water

Sauté for 5 minutes:

1 tsp. sesame oil
1¹/₂ onions, chopped
¹/₂ cup celery, chopped
2 cloves garlic, minced

Add and cook until soft:

1 Tbsp. barley malt syrup
2-3 tsp. curry powder
1 tsp. chili powder
¹/₂ tsp. ground coriander
¹/₄ tsp. cayenne

Drain lentils and add stock to vegetables, simmer 5 minutes. Add lentils and simmer 10 minutes. Serve over brown rice or couscous with side dishes of raisins, chopped green onions, shredded carrots and Ginger Pear Chutney (page 157)

Lentil Bulghur Loaf

6 servings

Wash and drain:
  1 cup lentils

Combine in pan with:
  3 cups water
  1 bay leaf
  1 tsp. oregano
  1 tsp. thyme

Bring to a boil, reduce heat, cover and simmer 35 minutes or until lentils are tender and liquid is absorbed. If lentils become dry, add a little more water.

In a small pan, bring to a boil 1 cup water.

Stir in and simmer for 1 minute:
  3/4 cup bulghur

Remove from heat, cover and let stand 20 minutes, until water is absorbed.

Simmer in small skillet:
  3 Tbsp. water
  1 cup onions, chopped
  1/2 cup celery, chopped
  3 cloves garlic, minced

Mix together the cooked lentils, the bulghur, the vegetables and:
  1/2 cup raw rolled oats
  2 Tbsp. soy sauce
  1/4 cup minced parsley
  juice of a half a lemon

Press into an oiled loaf pan, cover with foil. Bake at 350° for 40 to 50 minutes. Let loaf rest for 15 minutes, then slice.

Spicy Lentil Patties

12 patties

Rinse lentils and combine:
   1 cup lentils
   3 cups water

Bring to a boil, reduce heat, add:
   1 tsp. curry powder
   pinch of salt
   1 tsp. coriander
   1 tsp. cumin

Cover pan and cook 35-45 minutes until tender. Set aside with lid on.

Heat a skillet and sauté:
   1 tsp. olive oil
   ¼ cup carrot, chopped fine
   2 cloves garlic, chopped
   1 large onion, chopped

Lentils should absorb remaining liquid; if not, drain. Mash lentils, mix with sautéed vegetables and:
   1½ cups whole grain bread crumbs

Crumbs can be made by putting broken pieces of bread into a blender and blend a few seconds.

Mix in:
   2 Tbsp. wheat flour
   2 Tbsp. tomato paste mixed with 1 Tbsp soy sauce

Form into balls and flatten into patties. Place on an oiled baking sheet in a 350° oven. Bake 20 minutes, turn over and bake 20 minutes more.

Oat Mushroom Patties

20 patties

Bring to a boil in a 2 quart saucepan:
4 cups water or vegetable stock

Add and cook until soft:
¹/₂ cup onion, diced small
¹/₂ cup carrots, diced small
³/₄ lb. fresh mushrooms, diced

Add:
¹/₄ cup soy sauce
¹/₃ cup nutritional yeast
2 cloves garlic, minced
1 tsp. oregano
1 tsp. thyme
¹/₂ tsp. marjoram

Add 1 cup at a time, letting oats sink in, then stirring:
5 cups rolled oats

Cook for 5 minutes until mixture is thick at the bottom of the pot. Cover, set aside for 15 minutes, as it continues to thicken. Cool and shape into patties. Place on an oiled cookie sheet. Bake at 350° for 40 minutes, turning after 20 minutes.

Serve hot in buns or cold in sandwiches with lettuce and mayonnaise.

Tofu Meatless Loaf

6 servings

Crumble and mash:

1¹/₂ lb. tofu

Mix with tofu in a bowl:

1 cup whole grain bread crumbs
¹/₂ cup rolled oats
¹/₂ cup parsley, chopped fine
¹/₂ cup ketchup
2 Tbsp. Dijon mustard
¹/₂ tsp. garlic powder
¹/₂ tsp. thyme
1 large onion, chopped fine
1 medium green pepper, chopped fine

Press into an oiled loaf pan. Bake at 350° for 1 hour. Let cool 10 minutes before removing from pan to slice.

Vegetable Chop Suey

6 servings

Stir fry over medium heat a few minutes:

1 Tbsp. sesame oil
1 medium onion
1" fresh ginger
2 cloves garlic, minced
1/2 cup cabbage, sliced

Add to pan, then cover and cook 5 minutes:

1 medium carrot, sliced thinly
1 cup broccoli flowerets
1 green sweet pepper, diced
1 stalk celery, thinly sliced on the diagonal
3 cups vegetable stock or water
1/2 lb. tofu, in half inch cubes

Stir together:

2 Tbsp. cornstarch
1/4 cup cold water

Add to vegetables and stir until thickened. Stir in:

2 Tbsp. soy sauce
1 cup mung bean sprouts

Top with:

1-7 oz. can water chestnuts, sliced

Serve over brown rice.

Vegetable Pizza
with Whole Wheat Crust

6 servings

Mix together for crust:
> **1 Tbsp. dry yeast**
> **¼ cup warm water**

Let stand for 5 minutes, then add:
> **¾ cup water**
> **1 tsp. olive oil**
> **¼ cup cornmeal**
> **1½ cups whole wheat flour**
> **1½ cups whole wheat pastry flour**

Knead dough for 5 minutes until smooth and elastic. Cover and let rise 1 hour. Oil a cookie sheet and roll out pizza dough onto sheet. Push sides up for edges of crust.

Spread lightly with:
> **a thin layer of a low salt tomato sauce**

Sprinkle with:
> **1 tsp. each basil and oregano**

Simmer for 5 minutes:
> **3 Tbsp. water**
> **2 sliced onions**
> **1 sliced green pepper**
> **1 cup mushrooms**

Spread vegetables on top of pizza. Heat oven to 400° and bake pizza for 20-25 minutes.

Vegetarian Chili

8 servings

Wash, drain, cover and soak overnight:

2 cups kidney beans
¹/₂ cup pinto beans

Rinse beans, bring to a boil with:

7 cups water

Reduce heat, cover and cook 1 to 1¹/₂ hours until soft.

Heat a large pan and sauté:

2 tsp. olive oil
3 cloves garlic, crushed
1¹/₂ cups onion, chopped
1 cup celery, chopped
1¹/₂ cup carrots, chopped

When onions are almost tender add:

¹/₂ cup green pepper, chopped

Cook a few minutes more. Add

2 cups low salt tomato sauce
juice of 1 lemon
2 tsp. ground cumin
2 tsp. basil
2 tsp. chili powder
1 tsp. thyme
¹/₄ tsp. cayenne

Add:

the cooked beans
1 cup raw bulghur

Cook slowly for 10 minutes. Serve with a salad.

Vegetarian Lasagne

6 servings

Soak for 15 minutes in ¹/₂ cup hot water:
   ¹/₂ cup texturized vegetable protein (TVP)

Cook according to directions:
   ¹/₂ lb. whole wheat lasagna noodles

Mash in a large bowl:
   1 lb. firm tofu
   2 cloves garlic, chopped
   1 onion, chopped

Add to tofu:
   1 cup fresh mushrooms
   ¹/₂ lb. kale, steamed, chopped
   1 tsp. oregano
   ¹/₂ tsp. basil
   ¹/₂ tsp. thyme

Have ready:
   1-32 oz. jar tomato sauce
   2 cups steamed broccoli

Begin layering: place 3 noodles on the bottom of a lightly oiled 9" x 13" pan. Spread on a third of the tofu mixture. Cover with half the tomato sauce, the broccoli and some of the TVP. Continue layering noodles, tofu mixture, TVP and sauce, ending with noodles. Preheat oven to 350° and bake lasagne for 30 minutes.

ACCOMPANIMENTS

Barbecue Sauce

Makes 2 pints

Heat pan, add oil and sauté onion until tender.

1 tsp. oil
1 large onion, diced

Add to pan:

2 cups tomato puree (16 oz. can)
1-6 oz. can low salt tomato paste
1-6 oz. can water
¼ cup molasses
2 Tbsp. soy sauce
2 Tbsp. lemon juice
1 tsp. allspice
1 tsp. cayenne

Bring to a boil, then reduce heat to very low and cook uncovered an hour or more until thickness desired. Stir in:

2 Tbsp. lemon juice

Cook a few minutes more. Keep in refrigerator.

Brown Rice

4 servings

Wash in a saucepan of cool water, then drain thoroughly:

1 cup short grain brown rice

Put pan on medium heat and stir constantly until the rice dries, about one minute.

Add:

3 cups water

Bring to a boil, cover and simmer about 40 minutes, until the rice is soft but retains a hint of crunchiness. Do not overcook. If any water remains, drain it off.

Ginger Pear Chutney

Have ready:

3 lb. firm fresh pears (about 6 large)
2 cups brown rice syrup
1 green pepper, chopped small
2 cloves garlic, chopped small
2 jalapeño peppers, chopped small
2 Tbsp. fresh ginger, chopped
1 cup onions, chopped small
1 cup apple juice
1 cup apple cider vinegar
$^1/_2$ cup raisins
1 tsp. salt
1 tsp. allspice
juice of 1 lemon
rind of 1 lemon, finely shredded

Peel, core and chop the pears. Combine all ingredients in a large heavy-bottomed pan. Bring to a boil, then reduce heat to low and cook, uncovered, for about 2 hours. Stir frequently so it does not stick or scorch. It will thicken as it cooks. Pack while hot in small sterilized jars.

Mother Nature's Apple Butter

Makes 3 pints

Wash, core and cut up but do not peel:
   4 lb. apples

Place in large kettle with:
   3 cups apple juice or cider

Cover, bring to a boil on medium high heat, then reduce heat to low and simmer until apples are soft, 35-40 minutes, stirring occasionally. Put through a food mill or press through a sieve, discarding skins. Return fruit pulp to kettle, stir in:
   2 tsp. cinnamon
   1 tps. allspice
   $^1/_2$ tsp. ground cloves

Cook slowly 1 to 2 hours, stirring from time to time as it thickens. Pack in hot sterile jars or keep refrigerated.

Mushroom Gravy

Serve over mashed potatoes or cooked noodles.

Heat a skillet and sauté for 2 minutes:
1 cup fresh mushrooms, diced
1 tsp. sesame oil

Set mushrooms aside.

Mix and cook over medium heat until thick, whisking to avoid lumps:
2 cups cold water
2 Tbsp. cornstarch

Add mushrooms to sauce and stir in:
2-3 Tbsp. soy sauce

Cook until bubbling.

DESSERTS

Apple Bread Pudding

6 servings

Cut bread into 1" cubes. Place in a bowl:

3 cups whole wheat bread cubes, firmly packed
¹/₂ cup currants

Pour over the bread and soak 15 minutes:

1¹/₂ cups apple juice

Mix with bread:

2 apples, cored and cut up
2 Tbsp. toasted sunflower seeds
1 tsp. vanilla
¹/₄ tsp. nutmeg
pinch of salt

Mix well. Place in a lightly oiled casserole dish. Sprinkle with cinnamon. Bake uncovered at 350˚ for 45 minutes. Serve warm or chilled.

All Natural Fruit Cake

Makes 2 loaves

Snip into small pieces with scissors:
   1 cup dried papaya
   1 cup dried apricots
   ¹/₂ cup dried pineapple

Combine with:
   ¹/₂ cup currants

Cover with:
   2 cups apple juice or cider

Bring to a boil, cover, turn off heat and let stand 15 minutes. Drain, saving liquid. Let cool. Prepare 2 loaf pans by cutting strips of waxed paper to line bottom and sides with paper overhang. Oil bottom of pans and oil paper.

Mix in a large bowl:
   3¹/₂ cups whole wheat pastry flour
   3 tsp. baking powder
   1 tsp. nutmeg
   1 tsp. cinnamon
   ¹/₂ tsp baking soda
   ¹/₂ salt
   ¹/₂ tsp. mace

Make a well in the center of the dry ingredients, add:
   1 cup liquid drained from fruit (add water to make 1 cup if necessary)
   ¹/₄ cup oil
   ¹/₂ cup maple syrup
   2 Tbsp. molasses
   1 tsp. vanilla

Stir together and divide mixture into prepared pans. Heat oven to 300° and place a large pan of hot water on bottom shelf. Bake cakes on middle shelf. After 1 hour remove water and lay a piece of foil loosely over cakes if they are getting brown. Bake 30 minutes more. Remove from oven and cool, remove from pans and strip off waxed paper.

Aduki Carob Brownies

Makes 24 brownies

Rinse in cold water and discard any shrivelled beans:
   1 cup dried aduki beans

Bring to a boil with:
   2 cups water
   1 cup apple juice

Cover, reduce heat and cook until beans are tender, adding more liquid if necessary (45 minutes under pressure, 2 hours in a covered kettle). Mash beans until creamy.

Blend into beans:
   1 cup whole wheat flour
   1 cup applesauce
   ¹/₂ cup carob powder
   ¹/₂ cup buckwheat flour
   ¹/₄ cup oil
   1 tsp. vanilla
   1 tsp. cinnamon
   ¹/₂ tsp. baking soda
   ¹/₄ tsp salt

Preheat oven to 350°. Spoon into a well-oiled 9" x 15" pan. Bake 25-30 minutes or until firm. Cut into squares.

Baked Apples

Have ready:
4 apples, core removed

Heat oven to 350˚. Cover bottom of pie pan with
¼ cup unsweetened apple juice

Place apples in pan, spoon onto each:
1 tsp. maple syrup

Bake uncovered for 35-40 minutes until soft.

Baked Pears

4 servings

Peel, cut each in half and remove core from:
4 firm pears

Place core side up on a lightly oiled baking dish. Mix:
1 tsp. vanilla
¹/₄ cup barley malt

Put a spoonful in center of each pear. Sprinkle with:
1 tsp. ground ginger
¹/₄ tsp. nutmeg

Pour into pan:
¹/₂ cup apple or pear juice

Bake pears at 350° for 20 or 30 minutes, until tender. Serve 2 halves on a plate, spooning pan juices over them.

Date Oat Squares

Makes 16 squares

Place in blender and pulverize:
2 cups rolled oats

Mix with:
1 cup whole wheat pastry flour
$^1/_4$ tsp. salt
grated rind of 1 lemon

Stir into oat and flour mix until crumbly:
$^1/_3$ cup barley malt
2 Tbsp. oil

Pat $^2/_3$ of the dough into an oiled 9" x 9" pan.

For topping, combine in saucepan:
$1^1/_2$ cups chopped dates
$^2/_3$ cup water
pinch of salt
$^1/_2$ cup barley malt
juice of 1 lemon

Simmer the fruit in water until soft. Mash with lemon juice, salt and sweetener.

Spoon the fruit topping on evenly, sprinkle remaining dough on top. Preheat oven to 350˚ and bake for 35-45 minutes.

Fruit Kabobs

12 kabobs

Have ready:

3 red pears or apples
1 honey dew melon
¹/₂ fresh pineapple

Mix for a marinade:

¹/₂ cup orange juice
¹/₄ cup water
1 Tbsp. lemon juice

Core pears or apples but do not peel. Cut into 1" chunks and marinate so they do not turn brown. Cut pineapple in cubes. Use a melon baller, or cut melon into chunks. Soak in juice mixture in the refreigerator until serving. Thread onto 7" wooden skewers. Arrange on platter or stick skewers into half a grapefruit.

Fruit Salad

Don't prepare too far in advance as apples and bananas may discolor.

Makes 4 cups

Peel and dice orange over the bowl to catch all the juices.
   1 medium red apple, diced
   ¹/₄ pound seedless green grapes, cut in half
   1 banana, sliced
   1 medium orange, peeled and diced

Mix well and serve.

Ginger Cake with Lemon Sauce

9 servings

Combine:

2 cups whole wheat pastry flour
2 tsp. powdered ginger
¹/₂ tsp. salt

Add:

¹/₄ cup molasses
³/₄ cup brown rice syrup

Dissolve and add last, beating as you add:

1 tsp. baking soda in
1 cup boiling water

Spread evenly into a well-oiled 9" x 9" pan. Bake in a preheated oven at 350° for 30-35 minutes until sides begin to draw away from edge of pan. Cool, cut into 9 squares. Serve topped with warm lemon sauce from page 172.

Lemon Sauce

Bring to a boil:

    $^1/_2$ cup water
    $^1/_2$ cup brown rice syrup

Mix together:

    1 Tbsp. cornstarch
    $^1/_4$ cup cold water

Add the boiling water to the cornstarch mixture slowly then return to pan and cook until thickened, stirring constantly.

Stir into sauce:

    2 Tbsp. lemon juice
    2 tsp. grated lemon rind

Orange-Banana Compote

Makes 2 cups.

Cut up orange over a bowl to catch juice. Mix fruits.

    1 medium orange, peeled, diced
    1 medium banana, peeled, sliced

Index